BLACKWELL'S
UNDERGROUND CLINICAL VIGNETTES

PEDIATRICS, 2E

BLACKWELL'S
UNDERGROUND CLINICAL VIGNETTES

PEDIATRICS, 2E

VIKAS BHUSHAN, MD
University of California, San Francisco, Class of 1991
Series Editor, Diagnostic Radiologist

VISHAL PALL, MBBS
Government Medical College, Chandigarh, India, Class of 1996
Series Editor, U. of Texas, Galveston, Resident in Internal Medicine &
Preventive Medicine

TAO LE, MD
University of California, San Francisco, Class of 1996

JOSE FIERRO, MBBS
La Salle University, Mexico City

HOANG NGUYEN, MD, MBA
Northwestern University, Class of 2001

**Blackwell
Science**

CONTRIBUTORS

Abby Geltemeyer, MD
University of Texas, Houston, Resident in Medicine & Pediatrics

Mae Sheikh-Ali, MD
University of Damascus, Syria, Class of 1999

Navneet Dhillon, MBBS
Government Medical College, Chandigarh, Class of 1997

Ashraf Zaman, MBBS
International Medical Graduate

FACULTY REVIEWERS

Thao Pham, MD
UCLA, Fellow in Allergy & Immunology

Sue Hall, MD
UCLA, Associate Clinical Professor of Pediatrics

© 2002 by Blackwell Science, Inc.

Editorial Offices:

Commerce Place, 350 Main Street, Malden,
    Massachusetts 02148, USA
Osney Mead, Oxford OX2 0EL, England
25 John Street, London WC1N 2BS, England
23 Ainslie Place, Edinburgh EH3 6AJ, Scotland
54 University Street, Carlton, Victoria 3053,
    Australia

Other Editorial Offices:

Blackwell Wissenschafts-Verlag GmbH,
    Kurfürstendamm 57, 10707 Berlin, Germany
Blackwell Science KK, MG Kodenmacho Building,
    7-10 Kodenmacho Nihombashi, Chuo-ku,
    Tokyo 104, Japan
Iowa State University Press, A Blackwell Science
    Company, 2121 S. State Avenue, Ames, Iowa
    50014-8300, USA

Distributors:

The Americas
Blackwell Publishing
c/o AIDC
P.O. Box 20
50 Winter Sport Lane
Williston, VT 05495-0020
(Telephone orders: 800-216-2522;
    fax orders: 802-864-7626)
Australia
Blackwell Science Pty, Ltd.
54 University Street
Carlton, Victoria 3053
(Telephone orders: 03-9347-0300;
    fax orders: 03-9349-3016)
Outside The Americas and Australia
Blackwell Science, Ltd.
c/o Marston Book Services, Ltd.
P.O. Box 269
Abingdon
Oxon OX14 4YN
England
(Telephone orders: 44-01235-465500;
    fax orders: 44-01235-465555)

Acquisitions: Laura DeYoung
Development: Amy Nuttbrock
Production: Lorna Hind and Shawn Girsberger
Manufacturing: Lisa Flanagan
Marketing Manager: Kathleen Mulcahy
Cover design by Leslie Haimes
Interior design by Shawn Girsberger
Typeset by TechBooks
Printed and bound by Capital City Press

Blackwell's Underground Clinical Vignettes:
    Pediatrics, 2e
ISBN 0-632-04571-X

Printed in the United States of America
02 03 04 05 5 4 3 2 1

The Blackwell Science logo is a trade mark of
Blackwell Science Ltd., registered at the United
Kingdom Trade Marks Registry

Library of Congress Cataloging-in-Publication Data
Bhushan, Vikas.
Blackwell's underground clinical vignettes.
Pediatrics / author, Vikas Bhushan. – 2nd ed.
    p. ; cm. – (Underground clinical vignettes) Rev. ed.
of: Pediatrics / Vikas Bhushan ... [et al.].
c1999. ISBN 0-632-04571-X (pbk)
1. Pediatrics – Case studies. 2. Physicians – Licenses –
United States – Examinations – Study guides.
    [DNLM: 1. Pediatrics – Case Report. 2. Pediatrics –
Problems and Exercises. WS 18.2 B575b 2002]
I. Title: Pediatrics. II. Title: Underground clinical
vignettes. Pediatrics. III. Pediatrics. IV. Title. V. Series.
    RJ58 .B48 2002
    618.92'00076–dc21

                                   2001004890

CONTENTS

ACKNOWLEDGMENTS

Throughout the production of this book, we have had the support of many friends and colleagues. Special thanks to our support team including Anu Gupta, Andrea Fellows, Anastasia Anderson, Srishti Gupta, Mona Pall, Jonathan Kirsch and Chirag Amin. For prior contributions we thank Gianni Le Nguyen, Tarun Mathur, Alex Grimm, Sonia Santos and Elizabeth Sanders.

We have enjoyed working with a world-class international publishing group at Blackwell Science, including Laura DeYoung, Amy Nuttbrock, Lisa Flanagan, Shawn Girsberger, Lorna Hind and Gordon Tibbitts. For help with securing images for the entire series we also thank Lee Martin, Kristopher Jones, Tina Panizzi and Peter Anderson at the University of Alabama, the Armed Forces Institute of Pathology, and many of our fellow Blackwell Science authors.

For submitting comments, corrections, editing, proofreading, and assistance across all of the vignette titles in all editions, we collectively thank:

Tara Adamovich, Carolyn Alexander, Kris Alden, Henry E. Aryan, Lynman Bacolor, Natalie Barteneva, Dean Bartholomew, Debashish Behera, Sumit Bhatia, Sanjay Bindra, Dave Brinton, Julianne Brown, Alexander Brownie, Tamara Callahan, David Canes, Bryan Casey, Aaron Caughey, Hebert Chen, Jonathan Cheng, Arnold Cheung, Arnold Chin, Simion Chiosea, Yoon Cho, Samuel Chung, Gretchen Conant, Vladimir Coric, Christopher Cosgrove, Ronald Cowan, Karekin R. Cunningham, A. Sean Dalley, Rama Dandamudi, Sunit Das, Ryan Armando Dave, John David, Emmanuel de la Cruz, Robert DeMello, Navneet Dhillon, Sharmila Dissanaike, David Donson, Adolf Etchegaray, Alea Eusebio, Priscilla A. Frase, David Frenz, Kristin Gaumer, Yohannes Gebreegziabher, Anil Gehi, Tony George, L.M. Gotanco, Parul Goyal, Alex Grimm, Rajeev Gupta, Ahmad Halim, Sue Hall, David Hasselbacher, Tamra Heimert, Michelle Higley, Dan Hoit, Eric Jackson, Tim Jackson, Sundar Jayaraman, Pei-Ni Jone, Aarchan Joshi, Rajni K. Jutla, Faiyaz Kapadi, Seth Karp, Aaron S. Kesselheim, Sana Khan, Andrew Pin-wei Ko, Francis Kong, Paul Konitzky, Warren S. Krackov, Benjamin H.S. Lau, Ann LaCasce, Connie Lee, Scott Lee, Guillermo Lehmann, Kevin Leung, Paul Levett, Warren Levinson, Eric Ley, Ken Lin,

Pavel Lobanov, J. Mark Maddox, Aram Mardian, Samir Mehta, Gil Melmed, Joe Messina, Robert Mosca, Michael Murphy, Vivek Nandkarni, Siva Naraynan, Carvell Nguyen, Linh Nguyen, Deanna Nobleza, Craig Nodurft, George Noumi, Darin T. Okuda, Adam L. Palance, Paul Pamphrus, Jinha Park, Sonny Patel, Ricardo Pietrobon, Riva L. Rahl, Aashita Randeria, Rachan Reddy, Beatriu Reig, Marilou Reyes, Jeremy Richmon, Tai Roe, Rick Roller, Rajiv Roy, Diego Ruiz, Anthony Russell, Sanjay Sahgal, Urmimala Sarkar, John Schilling, Isabell Schmitt, Daren Schuhmacher, Sonal Shah, Edie Shen, Justin Smith, John Stulak, Lillian Su, Julie Sundaram, Rita Suri, Seth Sweetser, Antonio Talayero, Merita Tan, Mark Tanaka, Eric Taylor, Jess Thompson, Indi Trehan, Raymond Turner, Okafo Uchenna, Eric Uyguanco, Richa Varma, John Wages, Alan Wang, Eunice Wang, Andy Weiss, Amy Williams, Brian Yang, Hany Zaky, Ashraf Zaman and David Zipf.

For generously contributing images to the entire *Underground Clinical Vignette* Step 2 series, we collectively thank the staff at Blackwell Science in Oxford, Boston, and Berlin as well as:

- Alfred Cuschieri, Thomas P.J. Hennessy, Roger M. Greenhalgh, David I. Rowley, Pierce A. Grace (*Clinical Surgery*, © 1996 Blackwell Science), Figures 13.23, 13.35b, 13.51, 15.13, 15.2.

- John Axford (*Medicine*, © 1996 Blackwell Science), Figures f3.10, 2.103a, 2.110b, 3.20a, 3.20b, 3.25b, 3.38a, 5.9Bi, 5.9Bii, 6.41a, 6.41b, 6.74b, 6.74c, 7.78ai, 7.78aii, 7.78b, 8.47b, 9.9e, f3.17, f3.36, f3.37, f5.27, f5.28, f5.45a, f5.48, f5.49a, f5.50, f5.65a, f5.67, f5.68, f8.27a, 10.120b, 11.63b, 11.63c, 11.68a, 11.68b, 11.68c, 12.37a, 12.37b.

- Peter Armstrong, Martin L. Wastie (*Diagnostic Imaging, 4th Edition*, © 1998 Blackwell Science), Figures 2.100, 2.108d, 2.109, 2.11, 2.112, 2.121, 2.122, 2.13, 2.1ba, 2.1bb, 2.36, 2.53, 2.54, 2.69a, 2.71, 2.80a, 2.81b, 2.82, 2.84a, 2.84b, 2.88, 2.89a, 2.89b, 2.90b, 2.94a, 2.94b, 2.96, 2.97, 2.98a, 2.98c, 3.11, 3.19, 3.20, 3.21, 3.22, 3.28, 3.30, 3.34, 3.35b, 3.35c, 3.36, 4.7, 4.8, 4.9, 5.29, 5.33, 5.58, 5.62, 5.63, 5.64, 5.65b, 5.66a, 5.66b, 5.69, 5.71, 5.75, 5.8, 5.9, 6.17a, 6.17b, 6.25, 6.28, 6.29c, 6.30, 7.13, 7.17a, 7.45a, 7.45b, 7.46, 7.50, 7.52, 7.53a, 7.57a, 7.58, 8.7a, 8.7b, 8.7c, 8.86, 8.8a, 8.96, 8.9a, 9.17a, 9.17b, 10.13a, 10.13b, 10.14a, 10.14b, 10.14c, 10.17a, 10.17b, 11.16b, 11.17a, 11.17b, 11.19, 11.23, 11.24, 11.2b, 11.2d, 11.30a, 11.30b, 12.12, 12.15,

12.18, 12.19, 12.3, 12.4, 12.8a, 12.8b, 13.13a, 13.18, 13.18a, 13.20, 13.22a, 13.22b, 13.29, 14.14a, 14.5, 14.6a, 15.25b, 15.29b, 15.31, 15.37, 17.4.

- N.C. Hughes-Jones, S.N. Wickramasinghe (*Lecture Notes On: Haematology, 6th Edition*, © 1996 Blackwell Science), Figures 2.1b, 2.2a, 3.14, 3.8, 4.3, 5.2b, 5.5a, 5.8, 7.1, 7.2, 7.3, 7.5, 8.1, 10.5b, 10.6, 11.1, plate 29, plate 34, plate 44, plate 45, plate 48, plate 5, plate 42.

- Thomas Grumme, Wolfgang Kluge, Konrad Kretzschmar, Andreas Roesler (*Cerebral and Spinal Computed Tomography, 3rd Edition*, © 1998 Blackwell Science), Figures 16.2b, 16.3, 16.6a, 17.1a, 18-1c, 18-5, 41.3c, 41.3d, 44.3, 46.8, 47.7, 48.2, 48.6a, 53.5, 55.2a, 55.2c, 56.2b, 57.1, 61.3a, 61.3b, 63.1a, 64.3a, 65.3c, 66.3b, 67.6, 70.1a, 70.3, 81.2a, 81.4, 82.2, 82.3, 84.6.

- P.R. Patel (*Lecture Notes On: Radiology*, © 1998 Blackwell Science), Figures 2.15, 2.16, 2.25, 2.26, 2.30, 2.31, 2.33, 2.36, 3.11, 3.16, 3.19, 3.4, 3.7, 4.19, 4.20, 4.38, 4.44, 4.45, 4.46, 4.47, 4.49, 4.5, 5.14, 5.6, 6.18, 6.19, 6.20, 6.21, 6.22, 6.31a, 6.31b, 7.18, 7.19, 7.21, 7.22, 7.32, 7.34, 7.41, 7.46a, 7.46b, 7.48, 7.49, 7.9, 8.2, 8.3, 8.4, 8.5, 8.8, 8.9, 9.12, 9.2, 9.3, 9.8, 9.9, 10.11, 10.16, 10.5.

- Ramsay Vallance (*An Atlas of Diagnostic Radiology in Gastroenterology*, © 1999 Blackwell Science), Figures 1.22, 2.57, 2.27, 2.55a, 2.58, 2.59, 2.63, 2.64, 2.65, 3.11, 3.3, 3.37, 3.39, 3.4, 4.6a, 4.8, 4.9, 5.1, 5.29, 5.63, 5.64b, 5.65b, 5.66b, 5.68a, 5.68b, 6.110, 6.15, 6.17, 6.23, 6.29b, 6.30, 6.39, 6.64a, 6.64b, 6.75, 6.78, 6.80, 7.57a, 7.57c, 7.60a, 8.17, 8.48, 8.53, 8.66, 9.11a, 9.15, 9.17, 9.23, 9.24, 9.25, 9.28, 9.30, 9.32a, 9.33, 9.43, 9.45, 9.55b, 9.57, 9.63, 9.64a, 9.64b, 9.64c, 9.66, 10.28, 10.36, 10.44, 10.6.

Please let us know if your name has been missed or misspelled and we will be happy to make the update in the next edition.

PREFACE TO THE 2ND EDITION

We were very pleased with the overwhelmingly positive student feedback for the 1st edition of our *Underground Clinical Vignettes* series. Well over 100,000 copies of the UCV books are in print and have been used by students all over the world.

Over the last two years we have accumulated and incorporated **over a thousand "updates"** and improvements suggested by you, our readers, including:

- many additions of specific boards and wards testable content

- deletions of redundant and overlapping cases

- reordering and reorganization of all cases in both series

- a new master index by case name in each Atlas

- correction of a few factual errors

- diagnosis and treatment updates

- addition of 5–20 new cases in every book

- and the addition of clinical exam photographs within *UCV— Anatomy*

And most important of all, the second edition sets now include two brand new **COLOR ATLAS** supplements, one for each Clinical Vignette series.

- The *UCV–Basic Science Color Atlas* (*Step 1*) includes over 250 color plates, divided into gross pathology, microscopic pathology (histology), hematology, and microbiology (smears).

- The *UCV–Clinical Science Color Atlas* (*Step 2*) has over 125 color plates, including patient images, dermatology, and funduscopy.

Each atlas image is descriptively captioned and linked to its corresponding Step 1 case, Step 2 case, and/or Step 2 MiniCase.

How Atlas Links Work:

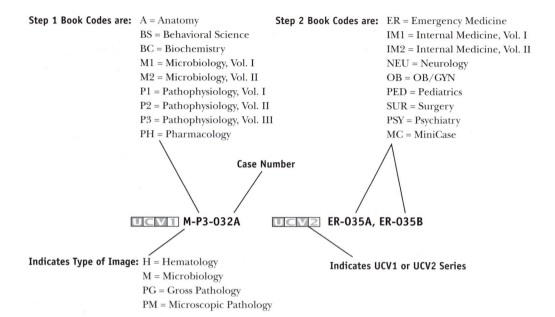

Step 1 Book Codes are:
A = Anatomy
BS = Behavioral Science
BC = Biochemistry
M1 = Microbiology, Vol. I
M2 = Microbiology, Vol. II
P1 = Pathophysiology, Vol. I
P2 = Pathophysiology, Vol. II
P3 = Pathophysiology, Vol. III
PH = Pharmacology

Step 2 Book Codes are:
ER = Emergency Medicine
IM1 = Internal Medicine, Vol. I
IM2 = Internal Medicine, Vol. II
NEU = Neurology
OB = OB/GYN
PED = Pediatrics
SUR = Surgery
PSY = Psychiatry
MC = MiniCase

Case Number

UCV1 M-P3-032A   UCV2 ER-035A, ER-035B

Indicates Type of Image:
H = Hematology
M = Microbiology
PG = Gross Pathology
PM = Microscopic Pathology

Indicates UCV1 or UCV2 Series

- If the Case number (032, 035, etc.) is not followed by a letter, then there is only one image. Otherwise A, B, C, D indicate up to 4 images.

   Bold Faced Links: In order to give you access to the largest number of images possible, we have chosen to cross link the Step 1 and 2 series.

- If the link is bold-faced this indicates that the link is direct (i.e. Step 1 Case with the Basic Science Step 1 Atlas link).

- If the link is not bold-faced this indicates that the link is indirect (Step 1 case with Clinical Science Step 2 Atlas link or vice versa).

   We have also implemented a few structural changes upon your request:

- Each current and future edition of our popular *First Aid for the USMLE Step 1* (Appleton & Lange/McGraw-Hill) and *First Aid for the USMLE Step 2* (Appleton & Lange/McGraw-Hill) book will be linked to the corresponding UCV case.

- We eliminated UCV → First Aid links as they frequently become out of date, as the *First Aid* books are revised yearly.

- The Color Atlas is also specially designed for quizzing—captions are descriptive and do not give away the case name directly.

New "MiniCases" replace the previous "Associated Diseases." There are now over **350 unique MiniCases** distributed throughout the *Step 2 Clinical* series, selected based on recent USMLE recollections.

We hope the updated UCV series will remain a unique and well-integrated study tool that provides compact clinical correlations to basic science information. They are designed to be easy and fun (comparatively) to read, and helpful for both licensing exams and the wards.

We invite your corrections and suggestions for the fourth edition of these books. For the first submission of each factual correction or new vignette that is selected for inclusion in the fourth edition, you will receive a personal acknowledgment in the revised book. If you submit over 20 high-quality corrections, additions or new vignettes we will also consider **inviting you to become a "Contributor" on the book of your choice**. If you are interested in becoming a potential "Contributor" or "Author" on a future UCV book, or working with our team in developing additional books, please also e-mail us your CV/resume.

We prefer that you submit corrections or suggestions via electronic mail to **UCVteam@yahoo.com**. Please include "Underground Vignettes" as the subject of your message. If you do not have access to e-mail, use the following mailing address: Blackwell Publishing, Attn: UCV Editors, 350 Main Street, Malden, MA 02148, USA.

Vikas Bhushan
Vishal Pall
Tao Le
October 2001

HOW TO USE THIS BOOK

This series was originally developed to address the increasing number of clinical vignette questions on medical examinations, including the USMLE Step 1 and Step 2. It is also designed to supplement and complement the popular *First Aid for the USMLE Step 1* (Appleton & Lange/McGraw Hill) and *First Aid for the USMLE Step 2* (Appleton & Lange/McGraw Hill).

Each UCV 2 book uses a series of approximately 50 **"supra-prototypical" cases as a way to condense testable facts and associations**. The clinical vignettes in this series are designed to give added emphasis to pathogenesis, epidemiology, management and complications. They also contain relevant extensive B/W imaging plates within each book. Additionally, each UCV2 book contains approximately 30 to 60 "MiniCases" that focus on presenting only the key facts for that disease in a tightly edited fashion.

Although each case tends to present all the signs, symptoms, and diagnostic findings for a particular illness, **patients generally will not present with such a "complete" picture either clinically or on a medical examination**. Cases are not meant to simulate a potential real patient or an exam vignette. All the **boldfaced "buzzwords" are for learning purposes** and are not necessarily expected to be found in any one patient with the disease.

Definitions of selected important terms are placed within the vignettes in (SMALL CAPS) in parentheses. Other parenthetical remarks often refer to the pathophysiology or mechanism of disease. The format should also help students learn to present cases succinctly during oral "bullet" presentations on clinical rotations. The cases are meant to serve as a condensed review, not as a primary reference. The information provided in this book has been prepared with a great deal of thought and careful research. This book should not, however, be considered as your sole source of information. Corrections, suggestions and submissions of new cases are encouraged and will be acknowledged and incorporated when appropriate in future editions.

ABBREVIATIONS

5-ASA	5-aminosalicylic acid
ABGs	arterial blood gases
ABVD	adriamycin/bleomycin/vincristine/dacarbazine
ACE	angiotensin-converting enzyme
ACTH	adrenocorticotropic hormone
ADH	antidiuretic hormone
AFP	alpha fetal protein
AI	aortic insufficiency
AIDS	acquired immunodeficiency syndrome
ALL	acute lymphocytic leukemia
ALT	alanine transaminase
AML	acute myelogenous leukemia
ANA	antinuclear antibody
ARDS	adult respiratory distress syndrome
ASD	atrial septal defect
ASO	anti-streptolysin O
AST	aspartate transaminase
AV	arteriovenous
BE	barium enema
BP	blood pressure
BUN	blood urea nitrogen
CAD	coronary artery disease
CALLA	common acute lymphoblastic leukemia antigen
CBC	complete blood count
CHF	congestive heart failure
CK	creatine kinase
CLL	chronic lymphocytic leukemia
CML	chronic myelogenous leukemia
CMV	cytomegalovirus
CNS	central nervous system
COPD	chronic obstructive pulmonary disease
CPK	creatine phosphokinase
CSF	cerebrospinal fluid
CT	computed tomography
CVA	cerebrovascular accident
CXR	chest x-ray
DIC	disseminated intravascular coagulation
DIP	distal interphalangeal
DKA	diabetic ketoacidosis
DM	diabetes mellitus
DTRs	deep tendon reflexes
DVT	deep venous thrombosis

EBV	Epstein–Barr virus
ECG	electrocardiography
Echo	echocardiography
EF	ejection fraction
EGD	esophagogastroduodenoscopy
EMG	electromyography
ERCP	endoscopic retrograde cholangiopancreatography
ESR	erythrocyte sedimentation rate
FEV	forced expiratory volume
FNA	fine needle aspiration
FTA-ABS	fluorescent treponemal antibody absorption
FVC	forced vital capacity
GFR	glomerular filtration rate
GH	growth hormone
GI	gastrointestinal
GM-CSF	granulocyte macrophage colony stimulating factor
GU	genitourinary
HAV	hepatitis A virus
hcG	human chorionic gonadotrophin
HEENT	head, eyes, ears, nose, and throat
HIV	human immunodeficiency virus
HLA	human leukocyte antigen
HPI	history of present illness
HR	heart rate
HRIG	human rabies immune globulin
HS	hereditary spherocytosis
ID/CC	identification and chief complaint
IDDM	insulin-dependent diabetes mellitus
Ig	immunoglobulin
IGF	insulin-like growth factor
IM	intramuscular
JVP	jugular venous pressure
KUB	kidneys/ureter/bladder
LDH	lactate dehydrogenase
LES	lower esophageal sphincter
LFTs	liver function tests
LP	lumbar puncture
LV	left ventricular
LVH	left ventricular hypertrophy
Lytes	electrolytes
MCHC	mean corpuscular hemoglobin concentration
MCV	mean corpuscular volume
MEN	multiple endocrine neoplasia

MGUS	monoclonal gammopathy of undetermined significance
MHC	major histocompatibility complex
MI	myocardial infarction
MOPP	mechlorethamine/vincristine (Oncovorin)/procarbazine/prednisone
MR	magnetic resonance (imaging)
NHL	non-Hodgkin's lymphoma
NIDDM	non-insulin-dependent diabetes mellitus
NPO	nil per os (nothing by mouth)
NSAID	nonsteroidal anti-inflammatory drug
PA	posteroanterior
PIP	proximal interphalangeal
PBS	peripheral blood smear
PE	physical exam
PFTs	pulmonary function tests
PMI	point of maximal intensity
PMN	polymorphonuclear leukocyte
PT	prothrombin time
PTCA	percutaneous transluminal angioplasty
PTH	parathyroid hormone
PTT	partial thromboplastin time
PUD	peptic ulcer disease
RBC	red blood cell
RPR	rapid plasma reagin
RR	respiratory rate
RS	Reed–Sternberg (cell)
RV	right ventricular
RVH	right ventricular hypertrophy
SBFT	small bowel follow-through
SIADH	syndrome of inappropriate secretion of ADH
SLE	systemic lupus erythematosus
STD	sexually transmitted disease
TFTs	thyroid function tests
tPA	tissue plasminogen activator
TSH	thyroid-stimulating hormone
TIBC	total iron-binding capacity
TIPS	transjugular intrahepatic portosystemic shunt
TPO	thyroid peroxidase
TSH	thyroid-stimulating hormone
TTP	thrombotic thrombocytopenic purpura
UA	urinalysis
UGI	upper GI
US	ultrasound

VDRL   Venereal Disease Research Laboratory
VS   vital signs
VT   ventricular tachycardia
WBC   white blood cell
WPW   Wolff–Parkinson–White (syndrome)
XR   x-ray

ID/CC A 2-year-old **girl** presents with **poor feeding** and **difficulty breathing**.

HPI She was born in a small town in the Rocky Mountains (**high altitude** predisposes) and was delivered at 28 weeks' gestation (more common in **preterm** infants). On directed questioning, her mother recalls that she had a transitory skin rash during the first trimester of her pregnancy (**rubella** predisposes).

PE VS: tachycardia; tachypnea. PE: **no cyanosis; bounding arterial pulses; wide pulse pressure; hyperdynamic** LV **impulse** displaced laterally; **continuous "machinery murmur"** noted at second and third left intercostal space lateral to sternal border.

Labs ECG: left axis deviation; LVH.

Imaging CXR: **increased pulmonary vascular markings**; enlarged left ventricle, left atrium, pulmonary arteries, and ascending aorta; the ductus arteriosus may show calcification. Echo: enlarged left atrium and ventricle. Angio: **increased oxygen saturation in the pulmonary artery** (diagnostic).

Pathogenesis Patent ductus arteriosus is failed closure of fetal communication between the pulmonary artery and aorta; commonly associated with maternal rubella and coxsackievirus infection, premature birth, and respiratory distress syndrome. The ductus normally closes as a result of increased oxygen tension during the first 48 hours of life (may take up to 5 days in term infants and up to 1 year in premature infants). The persistent communication between the descending aorta and pulmonary artery increases pulmonary blood flow in systole and diastole, causing pulmonary congestion and LV overload.

Epidemiology **Twice as common in females**; more common in infants born at high altitudes and in premature infants.

Management In the presence of respiratory distress syndrome, **treat heart failure** (diuretics, digitalis) and anemia. **Indomethacin**, a prostaglandin E_1 inhibitor, may stimulate ductus closure. **Surgery** consists of simple ligation (preferred), clipping, or division and may be considered in the absence of pulmonary hypertension. Administer **prophylactic antibiotics** with dental and surgical procedures.

PATENT DUCTUS ARTERIOSUS

Complications	If left untreated, there is a high risk of **left heart failure** (most common), subacute **infective endocarditis**, and **Eisenmenger's syndrome** (symptomatic **pulmonary hypertension** resulting from high pulmonary vascular flow; eventually leads to the development of a right-to-left shunt; manifests as right heart failure and cyanosis).
Atlas Link	⬛UCV1⬛ PG-A-006

MINICASE 296: CONGENITAL PROLONGED QT SYNDROME

A genetic defect of ion channels with variable penetrance
- presents with syncope in children precipitated by exertion
- ECG shows long QT at baseline with ventricular tachycardia during syncopal episodes
- treat with beta-blockers prophylactically or use drugs that can shorten the QT interval, such as phenytoin
- consider an implantable defibrillator for patients who have had a syncopal episode
- complications include sudden cardiac death

MINICASE 297: EISENMENGER'S COMPLEX

Chronic left-to-right shunting causes pulmonary vascular hyperplasia, pulmonary hypertension, and consequent shunt reversal
- usually seen with VSD, ASD, and PDA
- presents with dyspnea, hemoptysis, edema, and central cyanosis
- polycythemia
- ECG reveals RVH
- treat by heart-lung transplantation

ID/CC A 9-year-old girl presents with **shortness of breath** (DYSPNEA), mostly while running or playing, coupled with lightheadedness and **easy fatigability** (due to decreased cardiac output).

HPI Yesterday she complained of **severe chest pain** while skipping rope. She has no history of allergies, surgery, trauma, transfusions, hospitalizations, or major illnesses. Her vaccinations are up to date. The mother states that the child was born with **congenital rubella** (predisposing factor).

PE VS: normal. PE: **raised JVP** with prominent "a" wave; presystolic liver pulsation (increased venous pressure); palpable **RV heave**; crescendo-decrescendo (diamond-shaped) **systolic ejection murmur** preceded by click in left second interspace (pulmonary area); **single S_2** with **absent P_2** (S_4 heard when severe).

Labs CBC/Lytes: normal. ECG: right axis deviation; RV enlargement.

Imaging [A] CXR: **poststenotic dilated pulmonary artery** (1); note the relative size of the aortic knob (2). Other findings include

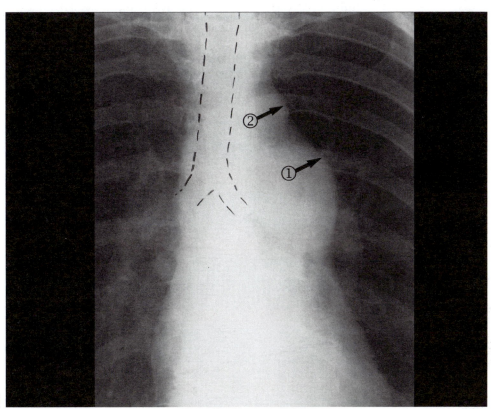

[A]

PULMONIC STENOSIS

diminished pulmonary vascular markings. Echo: RV enlargement; dome-shaped valve. Angio: transpulmonary gradient; RV pressure greater than systemic pressure.

Pathogenesis Pulmonic stenosis is a **cyanotic** congenital heart disease that is **idiopathic**, although some viral infections have been implicated (congenital rubella is a predisposing factor). In the **neonatal** period, patients may present with **cyanosis** (right-to-left shunt through patent foramen ovale); mild disease may be asymptomatic. In moderate to severe disease there may be exertional dyspnea, hypoxic spells, squatting episodes (more typical of tetralogy of Fallot), and even ischemic chest pain. It may be isolated but is more commonly associated with a patent foramen ovale or with other cardiac defects, such as VSD, ASD, and PDA. May be **valvular, infundibular**, or combined. Associated with Noonan's syndrome and malignant intestinal carcinoid.

Epidemiology Fifty percent of deaths occur within the first year of life unless a compensatory shunt (e.g., VSD, ASD, PDA) persists.

Management **Prostaglandin E_1** keeps the ductus arteriosus patent in neonates until surgery. **Balloon valvuloplasty** (mainly for isolated pulmonic stenosis) or surgical repair is required if the transpulmonary valve gradient exceeds 50 mmHg. **Emergent surgery** is indicated in acute right heart failure. RVH usually resolves after corrective surgery. Patients should be given antibiotic prophylaxis for **infective endocarditis** before dental and surgical procedures.

Complications Complications include **cardiac failure** (most common), sudden death (most frequently in infancy), low cardiac output, hypoxic spells, and arrhythmias. Postoperative complications include recurrence (mainly if surgery was done early) and pulmonary insufficiency.

ID/CC   A 3-year-old boy presents with **failure to thrive**.

HPI   The patient has **not been gaining weight** normally and tends to **tire easily** while playing.

PE   No cyanosis; **displacement of PMI to left**; sternal lift; harsh, **holosystolic murmur** at left sternal border.

Labs   ABGs: normal. ECG: LVH; RVH.

Imaging   [A] CXR: enlarged heart and dilated pulmonary vessels (1). Echo: moderate defect in the interventricular septum. Angio: pulmonary-to-systemic blood flow ratio is 1.5 to 1.0.

Pathogenesis   Ventricular septal defects can consist of isolated defects or of multiple anomalies. The opening is typically situated in the **membranous portion** of the septum; functional deficits depend on the size and status of the pulmonary vascular bed. The majority of patients have isolated large defects that are caught early in life. Two-dimensional echocardiography or color doppler examination can define the number and location of defects in the ventricular septum and detect other associated anomalies; hemodynamic and angiographic studies should be used as needed to determine the status of the pulmonary vascular bed and to further assess the anatomy. Five to ten percent of patients with moderate VSD and left-to-right shunt develop RV outflow obstruction. Incompetence of the aortic valve is also observed in approximately 5% of patients.

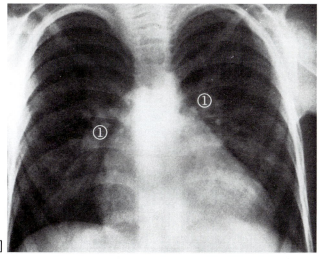

[A]

VENTRICULAR SEPTAL DEFECT

This results from insufficient cusp tissue or prolapse of the cusp through the interventricular defect. Aortic regurgitation then complicates and dominates the clinical course of these patients.

Epidemiology　VSD is the **most common congenital heart disorder**, accounting for approximately 30% of all congenital cardiac lesions.

Management　Patients with large VSDs (large left-to-right shunt), CHF, or pulmonary hypertension must undergo **surgical correction**. If corrected early, pulmonary vascular disease can be prevented. Surgery typically is not recommended for patients with small or moderate-sized defects and normal pulmonary arterial pressure.

Complications　A VSD may close spontaneously (if small), but CHF and death may also result. Eisenmenger's syndrome may develop; aortic regurgitation and infective endocarditis have also been observed.

Atlas Link　U C V 1 　PG-A-008

ID/CC	An 8-year-old boy is seen for a low-grade fever and **facial rash**.
HPI	His brother had a similar rash a few days ago. He has not had hematuria (rule out poststreptococcal glomerulonephritis).
PE	VS: low-grade fever (38°C). PE: **multiple vesicles and pustules** over the face and behind the ears measuring about 5 mm in diameter; lesions coalesce at places and are covered by a **honey-colored crust**; preauricular and **superficial cervical lymphadenopathy**.
Labs	Gram stain of exudate from rash shows **gram-positive cocci in chains**; culture yields **group A β-hemolytic streptococci**. UA: normal.
Pathogenesis	The causative agent of impetigo is most commonly **group A streptococci** (90% *Streptococcus pyogenes; Staphylococcus aureus* causes bullous impetigo). Impetigo is the most common streptococcal skin infection that **predisposes to glomerulonephritis**.
Epidemiology	Impetigo is **highly communicable** and occurs predominantly among preschoolers. Outbreaks of pyoderma-associated nephritis can occur in families or may spread in communities. The frequency of acute glomerulonephritis following infection caused by a known nephritogenic strain is 10% to 15%. The nephritogenic strains associated with impetigo (types 2, 49, 53, 55–57, and 60) differ from the pharyngitis-associated nephritogenic strains (types 1, 4, 12, and 25).
Management	**Oral penicillin** is the drug of choice for impetigo and ecthyma. **Erythromycin** is used in penicillin-allergic patients. Oral dicloxacillin or cephalexin is indicated for staphylococcal impetigo.
Complications	Poststreptococcal glomerulonephritis, lymphadenitis, and cellulitis.

IMPETIGO

MINICASE 298: DIAPER RASH

Inflammatory skin conditions occurring in the diaper area, caused either directly or indirectly from the wearing of diapers

- the precise etiology is unclear but is believed to result from prolonged exposure of the skin to urine and feces, leading to irritant contact dermatitis, miliaria, intertrigo, candidal diaper dermatitis, and granuloma gluteale infantum
- diaper rash is the most common dermatitis found in infancy
- presents with a rash consisting of shiny erythema with or without scaling of the skin found on the prominent parts of the buttocks, medial thighs, mons pubis, and scrotum
- diagnosis is usually made on the basis of clinical observation
- treat contact dermatitis with changes in diapering habits, candidal dermatitis with topical antifungal cream with every diaper change, bacterial infections with antibiotics, and granuloma gluteale infantum with low-potency corticosteroids
- complications include secondary infection

MINICASE 299: ERYTHEMA INFECTIOSUM

Also called "fifth disease"

- viral exanthem caused by parvovirus B19
- most often seen in children
- presents with a "slapped-cheek" facial rash that spreads to the arms and legs
- serum IgM to B19 is diagnostic
- no treatment is needed
- complications include aplastic crises, particularly in sickle cell disease

Atlas Link: [U][C][V][2] MC-299

MINICASE 300: KAWASAKI SYNDROME

Acute multisystem vasculitis seen in children

- presents with fever, "strawberry tongue," desquamating rash, lymphadenopathy, and conjunctival infection
- treat with IV immunoglobulin and NSAIDs
- complications include coronary artery aneurysms

Atlas Link: [U][C][V][2] MC-300

MINICASE 301: PITYRIASIS ALBA

A common hypopigmented dermatitis that occurs primarily in school-aged children
- presents with flaky, hypopigmented, patchy dermatitis with fine scales involving the face, neck, or shoulders
- laboratory workup with KOH stain and Wood's lamp exam to exclude other causes
- lesions are self-limiting and resolve by adulthood

MINICASE 302: ROSEOLA INFANTUM (EXANTHEM SUBITUM)

Rash and fever occurring in children under 3 years caused by human herpesvirus 6 (HHV6)
- presents with fever followed by a rash taking the form of small, rose-pink papules and macules in a face-sparing distribution
- resolves spontaneously within 2 days

MINICASE 303: SCALDED SKIN SYNDROME

Skin infection caused by exfoliative toxin-producing strains of *Staphylococcus aureus*
- presents with fever, periorbital edema, an erythematous rash with centrifugal spread, and wrinkled "sandpaper skin" with epidermal sloughing provoked by stroking (NIKOLSKY'S SIGN)
- staphylococci may be observed on denuded skin surface
- treat with IV penicillinase-resistant antibiotics (dicloxacillin)
- complications include fluid/electrolyte loss and systemic toxicity

MINICASES: 301–303

ID/CC	A newborn is seen by a neonatologist for **ambiguous genitalia**.
HPI	Her mother reports that the infant is **lethargic** and **lacks strength to suckle** (due to salt wasting). The parents are healthy with no relevant personal or family medical history.
PE	VS: no fever; hypotension; tachycardia. PE: well developed and nourished but **dehydrated; enlarged clitoris** and **fusion of labia majora**.
Labs	CBC: normal. Lytes: **hyponatremia; hyperkalemia. Increased serum 17-α-hydroxyprogesterone** and urine **pregnanetriol**; serum **androstenedione** and urinary **17-ketosteroids** elevated; elevated serum ACTH; low cortisol; low aldosterone.
Imaging	XR, external genitalia (with contrast media): **urogenital sinus**. CT, abdomen: bilaterally enlarged adrenal glands.
Pathogenesis	Congenital adrenal hyperplasia (also known as **adrenogenital syndrome**) is an **autosomal-recessive** deficiency of metabolic enzymes (most commonly 21-hydroxylase) that results in the accumulation of substrate steroids (usually 17-α-hydroxyprogesterone) and a deficiency of normal adrenal steroids. It is usually recognized early in females by the characteristic genital ambiguity (due to virilization) and salt wasting. In males, it may present as excessive muscularity, acne, excessive height, precocious sexual characteristics, and deep voice.
Epidemiology	**21-Hydroxylase deficiency** is the most common form of congenital adrenal hyperplasia, accounting for 95% of cases. **Prenatal diagnosis** can be established in the first trimester by chorionic villous biopsy followed by HLA typing and in the second trimester by measurement of 17-OHP in amniotic fluid. Newborns can also be screened.
Management	Administer **cortisol** to suppress the hypersecretory adrenal gland, thereby preventing early epiphyseal closure and virilization. If salt wasting is also present (half of cases), replace **mineralocorticoids** as well. Correction of external genitalia (in several operations) via **plastic surgery** can be done later.

CONGENITAL ADRENAL HYPERPLASIA

ID/CC	A 5-month-old **female** infant is seen for **sluggishness, edema,** and persistent **constipation.**
HPI	She appeared **normal at birth** except for mild **jaundice** that cleared somewhat but has not completely disappeared.
PE	VS: hypothermia; bradycardia. PE: mild jaundice, **dry skin, brittle hair, thick tongue, hoarseness,** hypertelorism, **flattened bridge of nose,** muscular **hypotonia, umbilical hernia,** short limbs, large anterior and posterior fontanelle.
Labs	CBC: anemia. **Low T_4** and **elevated TSH.**
Imaging	CXR: cardiomegaly. XR, long bones: delayed epiphyseal development (bone age); epiphyseal dysgenesis; beaking of T12 or L1 vertebrae; wormian bones.
Pathogenesis	Thyroid hormone deficiency (known as cretinism in children) may be primary or acquired. Most cases result from hypoplasia or aplasia or from embryologic maldescent of the thyroid. Other causes include hypothalamic and pituitary defects; deficiencies in iodine transport, concentration, organification, and coupling; failure of peripheral conversion of T_4 to T_3; peripheral resistance to thyroid hormone; defective thyroglobulin synthesis; and deficiency of iodide (ENDEMIC CRETINISM). It may also be caused by exposure to phenylbutazone, iodides (present in expectorants), or sulfonamides or by excessive ingestion of cabbage by women during pregnancy.
Epidemiology	Affects approximately 1 in 4,000 newborns. Thyroid dysgenesis has a familial, summer-season, and **female predominance** and shows a higher incidence among Hispanics than among blacks or whites.
Management	A **newborn screening** test with TSH and T_4 should be done in the first months of life to detect early hypothyroidism and to prevent mental retardation. Treatment involves the administration of **levothyroxine** with periodic TSH and T_4 measurements.
Complications	**Mental retardation,** dwarfism, pathologic fractures, coxa vara, coxa plana, and iatrogenic hyperthyroidism.

HYPOTHYROIDISM—CONGENITAL

MINICASE 304: 17-ALPHA-HYDROXYLASE DEFICIENCY

A genetic defect of adrenal steroid synthesis with a deficiency of glucocorticoid and androgen production and congenital adrenal hyperplasia (from increased ACTH production)
- presents soon after birth with hypertension, hypogonadism, and absence of secondary sex characteristics in females and ambiguous genitalia or female pseudohermaphroditism in males
- hypokalemia, metabolic alkalosis, elevated glucocorticoid and mineralocorticoid intermediates, and low urinary 17-ketosteroids
- treat with glucocorticoid replacement, surgery and exogenous estrogens/androgens for sexual differentiation abnormalities

MINICASE 305: 5-ALPHA-REDUCTASE DEFICIENCY

An autosomal-recessive disorder of virilization
- presents with microphallia, cryptorchidism, and hypospadias
- decreased 5-alpha-dihydrotestosterone with normal testosterone level
- treat with dihydrotestosterone

MINICASE 306: KWASHIORKOR

Protein energy malnutrition
- presents with apathy, irritability, muscle wasting with preserved subcutaneous fat, soft pitting edema, brittle and discolored hair, skin lesions (erythema, epidermis peeling off in large scales), and abdominal distention with hepatomegaly
- hypoalbuminemia, low hematocrit, and electrolyte disturbances
- fatty infiltration of the liver, small heart, and GI mucosal atrophy
- treat with replenishment of calories through assisted enteral or parenteral nutrition, correct electrolyte balances
- complications include infection and life-threatening electrolyte disturbances

MINICASE 307: PRECOCIOUS PUBERTY

Onset of secondary sexual characteristics prior to age 8 in females and prior to age 9 in males

- causes include but are not limited to abnormal function of or tumor in the ovaries, adrenal glands, hypothalamus, and pituitary
- presents with early breast development, pubic hair growth, and early menarche in females and increased growth rate, pubic hair, and testicular development in males
- basal elevated LH and FSH concentrations, pubertal LH response in response to GnRH stimulation testing
- x-ray of the skeleton shows increased bone age, US/CT/MR of the abdomen and pelvis to evaluate for ovarian or adrenal mass, CT/MR of the hypothalamus and pituitary to identify mass lesions
- treat with removal of adrenal or ovarian mass, GnRH analogs
- therapy varies according to cause

MINICASE 308: RICKETS

Vitamin D deficiency most commonly due to lack of sun exposure or nutritional deficiency in children

- presents with poor skull mineralization (CRANIOTABES), costochondral thickening (RACHITIC ROSARY), kyphoscoliosis, varus deformity of legs, and tetany
- hypocalcemia
- radiologic alterations are most apparent at the epiphyseal growth plate (particularly of the radius and ulna), which is thickened, cupped, and hazy at the metaphyseal border owing to decreased calcification and inadequate mineralization
- treat with vitamin D, calcium, and phosphate supplements

Atlas Link: UCV2 MC-308

MINICASE 309: VITAMIN A DEFICIENCY

Nutritional or malabsorptive deficiency of vitamin A, which is necessary for maintenance of normal retinal function and epithelial tissue

- presents with night blindness, xerophthalmia, and hyperkeratosis
- serum vitamin A levels < 30 to 65 mg/dL in advanced deficiency
- treat with vitamin A (retinol) replacement

A malignant neoplasm of primitive retinal cells having both hereditary and nonhereditary forms, with the hereditary form showing a deletion on chromosome 13q

- presents with diminished visual acuity, eye pain, tenderness of the eye to gentle palpation, unilateral proptosis, and a white amaurotic "cat's eye" reflex on funduscopic exam
- cytogenetics show deletion on chromosome 13
- CT/MR of the orbit shows retrolental mass
- treat unilateral tumor with enucleation, bilateral or metastatic disease may need radiation and chemotherapy

Atlas Link: UCV1 PM-P1-073

ID/CC	A 15-month-old girl appears **lethargic** after 3 days of persistent **vomiting** and **watery diarrhea** with no mucus or blood.
HPI	The mother states that the child has also had a mild **fever** and **does not have an appetite**. Her vaccinations are complete and up to date.
PE	VS: **fever** (38.2°C); **tachycardia** (HR 130); tachypnea (RR 21); hypotension. PE: **lethargic**; skin and mucous membranes are **pale, cold, and dry**; child cries but **no tears** are produced; **anterior fontanelle depressed**; poor skin turgor; abdomen slightly tender to palpation, but no masses or peritoneal signs; rectal exam reveals heme-negative stool (watery diarrhea).
Labs	CBC: **leukocytosis with lymphocyte predominance**. BUN and creatinine elevated; **stool shows no leukocytes** (nonbacterial diarrhea); stool culture and ova/parasites negative. ABGs: metabolic acidosis. Lytes: hypokalemia. **ELISA** is positive (specific for rotavirus).
Imaging	CXR: normal. KUB: nonspecific small bowel loop dilatation.
Pathogenesis	The most common cause of gastroenteritis in children younger than 2 years is **rotavirus**. Infection is transmitted through feces (direct contact, contaminated food and drink).
Epidemiology	Rotavirus has a winter predominance.
Management	Most cases are treated with **oral rehydration**; for severe dehydration, IV rehydration is indicated. **Antibiotics** should be given for *Shigella* and invasive *Escherichia coli* (TMP-SMX, ampicillin), amebiasis (metronidazole), cholera (tetracycline), and *Clostridium difficile* (metronidazole); symptoms of salmonellosis may be prolonged with antibiotics. **Anti-motility agents are contraindicated** in children because they prolong excretion of bacteria, virus particles, and exotoxins. A liquid diet low in lactose, followed by a soft diet, should be used.
Complications	The most common complication and cause of death **is fluid and electrolyte imbalance** (hypovolemia, metabolic acidosis, hypokalemia); other complications include septicemia (suspect in the presence of high fever, hypothermia, and lethargy without dehydration), acute renal failure (from acute hypovolemia), paralytic ileus, carbohydrate intolerance, pneumatosis intestinalis, and perforation with peritonitis and shock.

GASTROENTERITIS

ID/CC	A 10-year-old boy is admitted with **massive vomiting of bright red blood** (HEMATEMESIS).
HPI	For 2 days, the child has been passing **black, tarry** (MELENA), **foul-smelling stool**. His parents disclose that he has had similar episodes in the past, during which he was hospitalized and given multiple transfusions. Directed questioning also reveals that he received an umbilical exchange transfusion at birth.
PE	VS: tachycardia; orthostatic hypotension. PE: ill-looking and anxious; cold extremities; marked **pallor**; no icterus or clubbing; no signs of chronic liver disease or ascites; massive **splenomegaly**.
Labs	CBC: severe **normocytic anemia**; mild leukopenia and thrombocytopenia (due to **hypersplenism**). LFTs: normal. Coagulation profile normal; normal protein C and S levels; endoscopy shows presence of **actively bleeding varices**.
Imaging	US, abdomen: splenomegaly with small reflective channels (suggestive of portal hypertension as cause). Doppler studies: **prehepatic obstruction of the portal vein. [A]** Splenoportogram (now done rarely): massive collaterals with an enlarged splenic vein (1) and a completely obstructed (nonvisualized) portal vein; contrast directed to the esophageal (2) and gastric (3) varices and inferior mesenteric vein (retrograde flow). **[B]** UGI: multiple serpiginous filling defects in the esophagus, typical of indentation by varices.
Pathogenesis	**Umbilical vein sepsis** due to umbilical catheterization is usually the cause of prehepatic obstruction of the portal vein in neonates. Portal vein obstruction can also occur as a result of a tumor compressing the portal vein, but such an occurrence in childhood is exceedingly rare. **Recurrent variceal bleeding** and **splenomegaly** without evidence of liver dysfunction are the hallmarks of this disease.
Epidemiology	Portal vein thrombosis is the leading cause of portal hypertension in children without evidence of cirrhosis.
Management	Stabilize patients with immediate IV fluids and blood transfusions for acute bleeds; perform emergent upper GI endoscopy to confirm variceal bleed. **Scleropathy**, propranolol, and

portocaval shunting can be used for long-term management of portal hypertension.

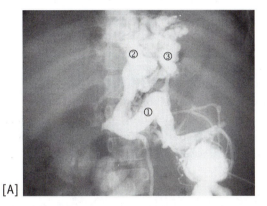

[A]

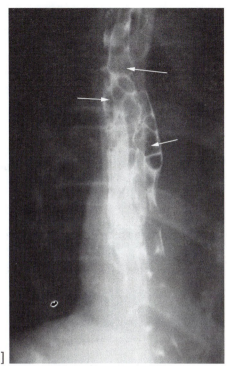

[B]

ID/CC	A 15-year-old girl presents with **jaundice**, spasmodic limb movements (CHOREA), and **behavioral changes**.
HPI	She has been performing poorly in school, and her mother notes that she has become increasingly labile and confused over the past few months.
PE	VS: normal. PE: jaundice; hepatomegaly; **[A] Kayser–Fleischer ring** (a brown band at the junction of the iris and cornea) seen on slit-lamp exam.
Labs	Elevated serum copper; low ceruloplasmin. LFTs: elevated AST and ALT; elevated bilirubin. Prolonged PT/PTT (signs of hepatic dysfunction); liver biopsy demonstrates **elevated parenchymal copper**. UA: elevated 24-hour copper level.
Imaging	MR, brain: cerebral atrophy with hypodensity of the putamen and globus pallidus.
Pathogenesis	Wilson's disease is an **autosomal-recessive** disorder of copper metabolism secondary to **defective biliary copper excretion**. This results in the abnormal accumulation of copper in the parenchymal cells of the liver, kidney, brain, and cornea. It most often manifests as **progressive hepatic dysfunction** that may be accompanied by **neuropsychiatric disorders**.

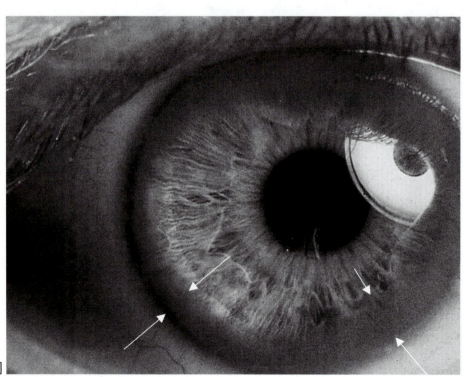

[A]

Epidemiology	Onset of disease is usually between the first and third decades of life.
Management	Chronic treatment with **copper-chelating agents** often halts the progress of the disease. **Liver transplantation** is indicated in cases of fulminant hepatic failure or progressive dysfunction despite chelation therapy.
Complications	Cirrhosis, hepatic coma, and death.

MINICASE 311: CRIGLER–NAJJAR SYNDROME

An inherited deficiency of glucuronyl transferase
- presents with severe jaundice and kernicterus causing seizures in neonates
- increased serum unconjugated bilirubin and low fecal urobilinogen
- treat with UV lamps and phenobarbital
- complications include irreversible brain damage from kernicterus

MINICASE 312: HIRSCHSPRUNG'S DISEASE

Congenital absence of parasympathetic myenteric ganglion cells in the rectum and sigmoid colon
- shows a familial tendency and is more common in males
- presents with abdominal distention and failure to pass stools in term infants
- rectal exam reveals an empty contracted rectum, with baby passing stools following the exam
- x-ray of the abdomen shows dilated colon proximal to the obstructing aganglionic segment
- rectal biopsy (pathognomonic) reveals aganglionosis
- treat by surgical excision of denervated bowel (narrowed segment)

Atlas Link: UCV1 PG-A-022

MINICASE 313: TRACHEOESOPHAGEAL FISTULA

A congenital fistulous connection between either the proximal or the distal esophagus and the trachea, associated with maternal polyhydramnios
- presents at birth with choking, cough, and vomiting with attempted feeding, a distended and tympanitic abdomen, and inability to pass a catheter into the stomach
- prenatal US shows excess amniotic fluid and no fluid in the stomach
- CXR shows feeding tube in blind esophageal pouch, gastric air bubble
- treat for aspiration pneumonia, keep pouch empty by constant suction, early surgical repair

ID/CC	A **2-year-old boy** presents with painless passage of **bright red blood per rectum** (HEMATOCHEZIA).
HPI	The patient's medical history is unremarkable, and his vaccinations are up to date.
PE	VS: **tachycardia** (HR 156); no fever. PE: conjunctiva and mucous membranes **pale; abdomen tympanic**; no palpable masses, hepatosplenomegaly, or peritoneal signs; heme-positive stool.
Labs	CBC: **anemia**; leukocytosis.
Imaging	Nuc: technetium scan demonstrates **heterotopic gastric mucosa** in the diverticulum. KUB: normal. **[A]** SBFT: a different patient with a typical diverticulum.
Pathogenesis	Meckel's diverticulum is caused by **persistence of the vitelline (omphalomesenteric) duct** (normally dissolves during the fifth to seventh week of intrauterine life). In children, it presents as **painless rectal bleeding**. Meckel's diverticulum may be found in an inguinal hernia (LITTRE'S HERNIA).
Epidemiology	The **most common congenital GI anomaly**. Predominantly affects males; characterized by the **rule of 2's**: affects 2% of population, 2 inches long, first 2 years of life, 2 feet from ileocecal valve, 2 types of epithelium (gastric and pancreatic).
Management	Achieve **fluid and electrolyte balance**; the definitive treatment is **surgical resection**. In the presence of peptic ulceration, the adjacent ileum is often involved and should be resected.

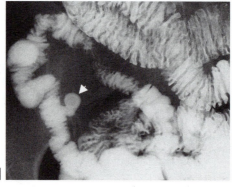

[A]

Complications	**Hemorrhage** (due to peptic ulceration; may be massive), **inflammation** (diverticulitis, appendicitis-like), **perforation, intussusception** (with intestinal obstruction), **umbilical drainage of ileal material** (omphaloenteric fistula, complete persistence of omphalomesenteric duct), **volvulus, foreign body obstruction,** and **intestinal obstruction** (due to fibrous remnants of the vitelline artery adhering to the umbilicus); rarely, leiomyoma, carcinoid, and adenocarcinoma.
Atlas Link	UCV1 PG-A-032

MINICASE 314: CLEFT LIP/PALATE

Due to failure of lip and palatal fusion during the first trimester, leading to unilateral or bilateral clefts of the soft and/or hard palate
- usually isolated, but may be associated with teratogens, a positive family history, or syndromes (trisomies 13 and 18, Pierre Robin)
- presents at birth with varied tissue involvement ranging from exclusive involvement of the lip and soft palate to bilateral involvement of the hard palate
- treat initially with modified feeding techniques and occupational therapy
- surgical correction during the first year of life, usually lip repair at 3 months and palate repair at 8 months
- if left untreated, may result in poor feeding, reflux, chronic middle ear effusions with hearing loss, speech difficulties, and dental or orthodontic problems

Atlas Links: UCV2 MC-314A, MC-314B

MINICASE 315: CLUBFOOT

Presents in infancy with plantar flexion of the foot at the ankle joint (EQUINUS), inversion deformity of the heel (VARUS), and forefoot varus
- treat with foot manipulation, serial casting
- surgery is required in > 50% of cases

Atlas Link: UCV2 MC-315

ID/CC A 4-year-old **white** male is brought to the pediatrician with complaints of **frequent, fatty, foul-smelling, bulky stools** (malabsorption) of about 3 months' duration, coupled with a **productive cough** (greenish, foul-smelling sputum), high fever, and difficulty breathing for the past day.

HPI He has a history suggestive of **meconium ileus** and rectal prolapse as well as **recurrent pulmonary infections** (inspissated mucus cannot be cleared from respiratory tract). He has also shown **failure to thrive** despite substantial caloric intake (due to malabsorption). A sibling has similar symptoms.

PE VS: **fever** (38.4°C); tachycardia; **tachypnea**. PE: **pale** and undernourished; **low weight and height for age**; nasal exam reveals **polyps** on left side (20% of cases); barrel-shaped chest; **dullness to percussion** in right lower lung field (due to pneumonia); crepitant rales with crackles and rhonchi; hepatomegaly.

Labs CBC: **anemia** (Hb 8.3) with micro- and macrocytosis (folate and iron deficiency due to malabsorption); **leukocytosis** with neutrophilia. Hyperglycemia (pancreatic endocrine insufficiency); hypoalbuminemia; **elevated sweat chloride** levels; **sputum culture yields *Pseudomonas***. PFTs: increased residual volume and total lung capacity. ABGs: hypoxemia.

Imaging **[A]** CXR: an older patient shows hyperinflation; ring shadows (suggesting bronchiectasis). **[B]** CT, chest: another patient with thick-walled, dilated bronchi in the left lower lobe from recurrent pneumonia.

Pathogenesis Cystic fibrosis (CF) is an **autosomal-recessive** disorder affecting the exocrine glands; it is due to a mutation of chromosome

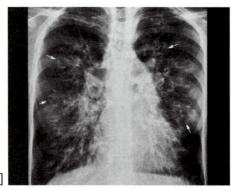

[A]

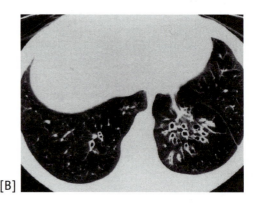

[B]

7q carrying the **cystic fibrosis transmembrane regulator (CFTR)** gene. The mutation produces alterations in chloride and water transport in epithelial cells, with secretion of abnormal mucus (thick and viscous) that plugs gland ducts (mostly in the pancreas and bronchi), leading to chronic pancreatitis and bronchiectasis. CF is characterized by recurrent URIs, lower respiratory tract infections (commonly with *Pseudomonas* and *Staphylococcus aureus*), lung scarring, and pneumothorax.

Epidemiology A common genetic disease in Caucasians, with an incidence of **1 in 3,500 whites**; 1 in 25 is a carrier of a mutation in the CFTR gene. **Median survival** is 29 years.

Management General management includes a **low-fat diet**, adequate hydration, vitamins, minerals (salt), and enzyme supplements. Steroid use is controversial; **recombinant human DNase** renders mucus less viscous (side effect is hoarseness). In the presence of **pseudomonal pneumonia**, give tobramycin with piperacillin, ticarcillin, or ceftazidime. **Lung transplantation** is an option but is costly and associated with a high rate of bronchiolitis obliterans. Prevention of lung infections includes **immunizations against *Pneumococcus* and influenza, chest physiotherapy**, postural drainage, antibiotics, and bronchodilators.

Complications Increased risk of GI tract malignancy, biliary cirrhosis, **pancreatic exocrine insufficiency**, gallstones, appendicitis, pulmonary fibrosis, exudative retinopathy, optic neuritis, diabetes, bleeding/coagulation problems, night blindness, osteomalacia, and azoospermia; in neonates, heat shock, rectal prolapse, and **meconium ileus** occur.

MINICASE 316: ALKAPTONURIA

An autosomal-recessive disorder of tyrosine metabolism
- presents with dark, blackened spots in the sclera and ear cartilage (OCHRONOSIS) and with pain and swelling of joints
- urine turns black if left standing
- treat arthritis with NSAIDs

ID/CC	A 6-year-old boy presents with progressive **mental retardation, diminished visual acuity**, and **deformity of the bones of his chest**.
HPI	The boy exhibits marked **developmental delay**. Two years ago he developed a **DVT** of the left leg (due to hypercoagulability).
PE	VS: normal. PE: **fair skin**; tall and thin with **long limbs** and abnormally long fingers (ARACHNODACTYLY); shuffling gait and mild **mental retardation** (due to recurrent cerebral thrombosis); fine hair and pectus carinatum; **glaucoma, cataracts**, and **lenticular dislocation** (ECTOPIA LENTIS); **malar flush**.
Labs	CBC/Lytes: normal. **Increased plasma methionine and homocysteine**. UA: **homocystinuria**.
Imaging	XR: generalized **osteoporosis**. **[A]** XR, spine: lumbar spine shows loss of bone density with vertebral collapse. **[B]** XR, spine: normal lumbar spine for comparison.
Pathogenesis	Homocystinuria is an **autosomal-recessive** disorder that is most commonly due to hepatic **cystathionine β-synthase deficiency**.

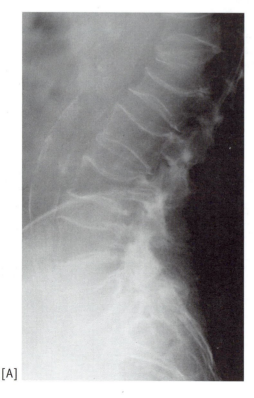
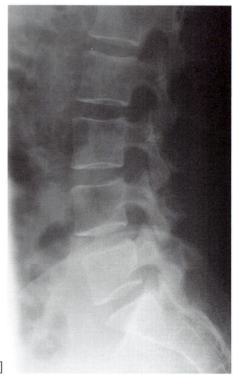

[A] [B]

It is clinically characterized by **recurrent thromboembolic episodes** (hypercoagulable state due to increased platelet adhesiveness in the presence of elevated homocystine levels) as well as by lens dislocation (myopia may precede ectopia lentis), cataracts, mental retardation, seizures, astigmatism, glaucoma, and a marfanoid body type.

Epidemiology   Rare.

Management   Treatment is mainly supportive. In approximately 50% of patients, **high doses of pyridoxine** diminish mental retardation if started early in infancy. If patients do not respond to pyridoxine, dietary **restriction of methionine** and **cysteine supplementation** are necessary.

Complications   Cerebrovascular accidents, MI, arteriosclerotic heart disease, renal and pulmonary embolism, retinal detachment, and fractures.

MINICASE 317: DOWN'S SYNDROME

The most common chromosomal disorder, due to trisomy 21
- higher incidence in advancing maternal age
- older patients with Down's syndrome are predisposed to Alzheimer's dementia
- presents as a developmentally retarded neonate with classic Down's facies (epicanthal folds, low-set ears, macroglossia), hypotonia, and simian crease
- karyotype reveals trisomy 21
- prenatal diagnosis is possible by chromosomal analysis of chorionic villous biopsy or amniocentesis and decreased levels of maternal serum α-fetoprotein levels
- treatment consists of social service support
- common complications include leukemia and heart disease

MINICASE 318: EHLERS–DANLOS SYNDROME

A group of genetic disorders of collagen synthesis with variable inheritance
- presents with hyperelastic skin, hyperextensible joints, and easy bruising
- skin biopsy shows large irregular collagen fibrils
- treatment is supportive
- patients are prone to dissection and aneurysm of the great vessels

GENETICS

ID/CC   A 10-year-old **mentally retarded boy** is brought to a physician by his parents because of bizarre, **self-destructive behavior**.

HPI   The boy frequently **bites his lips, fingers, and buccal mucosa**. Yesterday he attempted to put his hand in a fire. He has been **growth-retarded** since infancy. Last year he underwent surgery for bilateral **ureteral stones**. His maternal uncle had a similar disease and died of a self-inflicted head injury.

PE   VS: normal. PE: far below mental and physical standards appropriate for age; **choreoathetoid movements** of hands; lips and fingers have been bitten in multiple places; **spastic weakness and hyperreflexia** of lower limbs; tophi over extensor surfaces of elbows, knees, fingers, and toes.

Labs   Serum **uric acid levels markedly elevated** (HYPERURICEMIA). RBCs demonstrate **absence of enzyme hypoxanthine-guanine phosphoribosyltransferase (HGPRT)**. UA: uric acid crystals.

Pathogenesis   Lesch–Nyhan syndrome is an **X-linked recessive disorder** seen only in males. It is caused by a severe deficiency of HGPRT, an enzyme that retrieves hypoxanthine and guanine through salvage pathways for utilization in nucleotide synthesis. In the absence of this enzyme, hypoxanthine and guanine can be catabolized only through xanthine to uric acid, causing hyperuricemia and hyperuricosuria.

Management   **Allopurinol** controls uric acid crystalluria and the tendency toward stone formation. It also prevents development of gouty arthritis (which usually occurs after puberty). There is no specific therapy for neurologic symptoms, although gene therapy may be possible in the future.

ID/CC	A 4-year-old boy presents with **progressively more severe mental retardation** and hyperactivity with purposeless movements.
HPI	The child **developed normally for the first 2 to 3 months**. He is **fairer** than his siblings and, unlike them, has blue eyes and blond hair (due to albinism). He did not undergo screening for any congenital disorder.
PE	Severely mentally retarded with **fair skin, blue eyes**, and characteristic **"mousy" or musty odor**; neurologic exam reveals hypertonicity with hyperactive DTRs.
Labs	Guthrie test (bacterial inhibition assay method) positive; **plasma phenylalanine elevated** (> 20 mg/dL); plasma tyrosine normal; elevated urinary phenylpyruvic and o-hydroxyphenylacetic acid; tetrahydrobiopterin concentration normal. EEG: abnormal.
Pathogenesis	Phenylketonuria (PKU) is an **autosomal-recessive** disease that is due to deficient or absent **phenylalanine hydroxylase**, resulting in toxic accumulation of phenylalanine and its metabolites. Patients with this disorder have fair skin and blue eyes owing to the decreased availability of tyrosine for conversion into melanin. In maternal PKU, the persistent elevation of plasma phenylalanine concentration perfusing the heterozygous fetus during development increases the risk of mental retardation, heart defects, and prenatal growth delay.
Management	Give **diet formulas low in phenylalanine** and monitor serum levels. Diet should also have **adequate amounts of tyrosine. Avoid aspartame** (Nutrasweet), which is broken down by the body into phenylalanine. **Neonatal screening** is essential in preventing the development of mental retardation in affected children.

14 PHENYLKETONURIA (PKU)

ID/CC	A 10-year-old boy presents with **recurrent fatigue**, anxiety, nausea, **lightheadedness**, and **sweating** (due to hypoglycemia) that are precipitated by short periods of **fasting** or **exercise**.
HPI	His mother states that his **symptoms are relieved by eating**. She adds that her son also has a **bleeding tendency** (due to platelet dysfunction). Occasionally he complains of severe **pain and swelling of his big toe** (due to gout).
PE	VS: normal. PE: pale; **obese** with **"doll's face"**; no mental retardation; enlarged tongue (MACROGLOSSIA); **low weight for age**; tendon xanthomas; **purpuric spots on legs and arms**; abdomen distended; **marked hepatomegaly**; no splenomegaly; soft **tophi** on elbows and ears.
Labs	CBC: normochromic anemia. **Elevated blood lactic and pyruvic acid** (LACTIC ACIDOSIS); elevated serum uric acid (HYPERURICEMIA); hypophosphatemia; **hypercholesterolemia; hypertriglyceridemia; severe fasting hypoglycemia** (glucose < 40 mg/dL); prolonged PT and bleeding time; **IV galactose/ fructose does not raise blood glucose level** (not converted to glucose); IV glucagon is not followed by rise in blood glucose (GLUCAGON TOLERANCE TEST); **hepatic biopsy** reveals fatty liver with increased deposition of glycogen (glycogen-lipid droplets) and **absence of glucose-6-phosphatase.**
Imaging	US: diffuse hepatomegaly; **kidneys enlarged bilaterally.**
Pathogenesis	Von Gierke's disease is an **autosomal-recessive** glycogen storage disease (type I) caused by a **deficiency** of **glucose-6-phosphatase**; it is characterized by failure to convert glucose-6-phosphate to glucose, with resulting deposition of glycogen in tissues. Von Gierke's disease presents at birth or in the first year of life and involves the liver, kidneys, and intestine. There is **no skeletal or cardiac muscle involvement (since this enzyme is normally absent here).**
Epidemiology	Von Gierke's disease is the **most common glycogen storage disease.**
Management	Give **frequent, small meals** (high in carbohydrates and protein) to prevent hypoglycemia and ketosis; continuous overnight gastrointestinal tube feedings. Use probenecid and allopurinol for hyperuricemia. Portacaval shunts have not yielded encouraging results, with cirrhosis and hepatic encephalopathy as

frequent complications. Abdominal US or CT should be performed every 6 to 12 months, as patients are at **risk for hepatoma**.

Complications   Cardiac failure, cyanosis, convulsions, coma, hepatic adenomas and carcinomas, and liver cirrhosis.

MINICASE 319: GAUCHER'S DISEASE

An autosomal-recessive deficiency of the enzyme glucocerebrosidase frequently found in Jewish people of Eastern European origin
- presents with epistaxis, easy bruising, bone pain, and massive splenomegaly
- bone marrow biopsy reveals typical Gaucher cells (characterized by an eccentric nucleus and "wrinkled" cytoplasm with PAS-positive fibrillar inclusion bodies)
- deficient glucocerebrosidase activity in leukocytes is diagnostic
- treat with recombinant acid β-glucosidase

MINICASE 320: GLYCOGEN STORAGE DISEASES

Genetic defects of enzymes in the glycogen synthetic or degradative pathways
- present with organomegaly involving the liver, heart, kidney, or muscle
- hypoglycemia and exercise intolerance
- enzyme assay of tissue reveals deficiency
- treat with frequent carbohydrate-rich meals to ameliorate symptoms
- complications include lactic acidosis and growth retardation

---

MINICASE 321: KLINEFELTER'S SYNDROME

Also known as testicular dysgenesis, it is the most common cause of male hypogonadism
- presents with increased height, eunuchoid body habitus, gynecomastia, testicular atrophy, and impotence
- karyotype 47,XXY
- treat with androgen replacement

ID/CC A **4-year-old** white **male** is brought to the pediatrician with **pallor, fever, and joint pain** of several days' duration. Today he had an episode of spontaneous nosebleed (EPISTAXIS).

HPI The child has been complaining of **fatigue** and **bone pain** on and off for the past 2 months and has also had **repeated URIs** over the past 6 months.

PE VS: **fever** (38.3°C); tachycardia (HR 110). PE: mucous membranes and conjunctiva **pale**; epistaxis and gingival bleeding with minor pressure; **ecchymotic patches** on skin of legs and arms; generalized **lymphadenopathy; sternal tenderness** elicited on pressure; nontender **hepatosplenomegaly.**

Labs CBC/PBS: normocytic, normochromic **anemia** (Hct 24%); **leukopenia; lymphocytosis;** neutropenia; **thrombocytopenia** (40,000); **[A] numerous immature leukocytes (blast cells).** Increased serum LDH; increased serum uric acid (HYPERURICEMIA); **CALLA** (CD10) **positive, and terminal deoxynucleotidyl transferase positive** (marker of immature T and B lymphocytes;

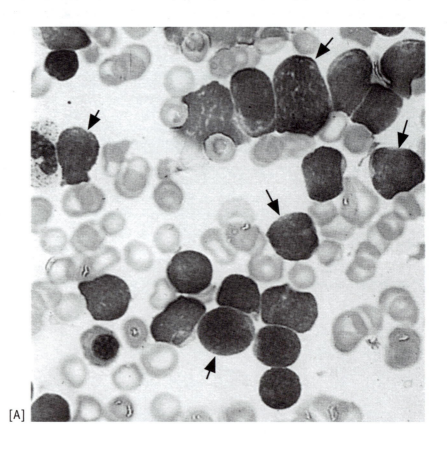

[A]

differentiates from nonlymphoblastic leukemia); bone marrow biopsy shows **sheets of malignant lymphoblasts** replacing normal marrow.

Imaging CXR: mediastinal mass seen (commonly secondary to lymphadenopathy or thymic infiltration).

Pathogenesis Acute lymphocytic leukemia (ALL) is a malignant proliferation of bone marrow lymphocyte precursors (LYMPHOBLASTS) with bone marrow infiltration. Radiation, alkylating agents, and benzene exposure are associated with increased risk. It is classified as types L1 to L3 (L1, childhood type; L2, adult type; L3, Burkitt's type) and may also be classified as B-cell (most common), T-cell, or small cell type. It is more commonly seen in **Down's syndrome**, in patients with ataxia-telangiectasia, in patients with chromosome 5 and 7 abnormalities, and in the twin siblings of patients with the disease.

Epidemiology ALL is the **most common pediatric malignancy**, followed by brain tumors. It constitutes 80% of all childhood leukemias and has a male predominance. **Most childhood leukemias are acute**.

Management **Combination chemotherapy** (daunorubicin, vincristine, prednisone, and asparaginase) is used to induce remission (normal PBS and bone marrow morphology; clinically asymptomatic) and consolidation (POSTREMISSION THERAPY). **Bone marrow transplantation** may also be considered. The vast majority of patients remit; most will not relapse. **Tumor lysis syndrome** may be prevented by using allopurinol and adequate IV hydration prior to chemotherapy. Treat infection with antibiotics, anemia with transfusions, and thrombocytopenia with platelet concentrates. Given the risk of CNS disease, LP should be performed to rule out malignant involvement.

Complications Sepsis (*Escherichia coli*, *Klebsiella*, *Pseudomonas*, *Candida*); meningeal, testicular, and mediastinal involvement (more common with T-cell type); spontaneous bleeding (if platelet count < 20,000); and relapse.

Atlas Links UCV1 H-P2-013A, H-P2-013B, H-P2-013C

ID/CC	A 4-year-old boy is admitted with a **high-grade fever**.
HPI	His mother reveals that he has a history of **recurrent episodes of high-grade fever and mouth ulcers**; these episodes occur at intervals of 3 to 4 weeks. In between, the boy remains well.
PE	VS: tachycardia; high-grade **fever**. PE: multiple aphthous ulcers; cervical **lymphadenopathy; no hepatosplenomegaly or sternal tenderness**.
Labs	CBC: **leukopenia; absence of neutrophils**; neutrophil counts recover completely over 2 weeks. Blood culture yields *Staphylococcus aureus*.
Pathogenesis	Cyclic neutropenia is characterized by **periodic wide fluctuations in absolute neutrophil count**. The disorder is attributed to a regulatory defect of stem cells.
Epidemiology	The disease is rare and is generally detected in childhood. There is usually a positive **family history**.
Management	Administer **parenteral antibiotics**; give **granulocyte colony-stimulating factor** to stimulate neutrophil production, shorten the duration of neutropenia, and help reduce the severity of symptoms and infections.

MINICASE 322: THALASSEMIA—BETA

Decreased synthesis of β-globin chains due to errors in the transcription and translation of mRNA
- occurs most commonly in persons of Mediterranean descent
- presents with pallor, failure to thrive, delayed developmental milestones, maxillary hypertrophy, and splenomegaly
- CBC shows anisopoikilocytosis, HbF 95%, HbA absent
- x-ray of the skull shows "hair on end" appearance of frontal bone
- treat with blood transfusions as required together with chelation of iron with desferrioxamine, splenectomy (for hypersplenism), bone marrow transplantation

CYCLICAL NEUTROPENIA

ID/CC	A 7-year-old **boy** is brought to an urgent-care clinic with an acutely **swollen and tender right knee** and a cut in his lip that has been **oozing blood** for the past day.
HPI	The child's **brother and maternal uncles died of bleeding complications**, and he has always had **easy bruising**. Yesterday he participated in a soccer game and fell several times.
PE	VS: normal. PE: small superficial laceration on inner aspect of lower lip that bleeds easily when touched with a cotton swab; knee swollen and warm to the touch with slight redness of skin; **multiple ecchymoses** on legs and arms.
Labs	CBC: mild normocytic **anemia. Normal bleeding time** (von Willebrand factor present); **PT normal; PTT prolonged; factor VIII:C level reduced**; factor VIII antigen normal.
Imaging	XR, knee: soft tissue swelling with intra-articular fluid (secondary to hemarthrosis).
Pathogenesis	Hemophilia is an **X-linked recessive** disorder associated with the absence or diminished activity of **factor VIII coagulant protein** (FACTOR VIII:C). Factor VIII:C levels of < 1% are labeled as severe disease; levels between 1% and 5% indicate moderate disease; and levels > 5% are labeled as mild disease.
Epidemiology	Hemophilia A (factor VIII deficiency) accounts for 80% of cases; hemophilia B (factor IX deficiency, also known as Christmas disease; clinically indistinguishable from hemophilia A) accounts for 15%, and hemophilia C (due to deficiency of factor XI) for 5%. The vast majority of patients have a **family history** of bleeding. Females are carriers and **males express the disease (X-linked recessive)**.
Management	Parenteral **factor VIII concentrates** are the mainstay of therapy. Since the active life of factor VIII is not more than 24 hours, repeated doses are usually needed. **Desmopressin** IV or nasal spray may be used in mild to moderate cases by stimulating the body's production of endogenous factor VIII. Repeated **blood transfusions** are frequently required. Give **ε-aminocaproic acid** prior to dental work. Avoid aspirin and contact sports.
Complications	Intra-articular, intracranial, or intra-abdominal bleeding as well as compartment syndrome and disabling joint disease may develop. Treated patients may develop inhibitors to factor VIII (which render exogenous factor VIII ineffective, causing refractory bleeding) and are at risk of acquiring HIV or hepatitis from multiple transfusions.
Atlas Link	UCV2 **PED-018**

HEMOPHILIA

ID/CC	A **5-year-old boy** presents with **recurrent abdominal and joint pain**.
HPI	Yesterday his mother also noticed **black stools** (MELENA; due to GI bleeding) and a **rash over his buttocks**. He has a **history of allergy** that includes atopic dermatitis in early infancy and intermittent asthma attacks. He suffered from a **URI 2 weeks ago**.
PE	VS: no fever; mild hypotension (BP 100/70); normal HR. PE: mild periorbital **edema; petechiae and palpable purpuric lesions** with **urticarial** features noted over extensor surfaces of **lower extremities** and **buttocks**.
Labs	CBC: mild leukocytosis; **normal platelets**. Elevated ESR. UA: **hematuria**; mild proteinuria. **Heme-positive stool; serum IgA increased**; kidney biopsy shows IgA and complement deposits; ANA negative.
Imaging	CXR/KUB: normal. US, kidney: normal.
Pathogenesis	Henoch–Schönlein (ANAPHYLACTOID) purpura is an **immune-mediated hypersensitivity vasculitis** characterized by inflammation and necrosis of small blood vessels (LEUKOCYTOCLASTIC VASCULITIS). It is idiopathic with an allergic component and presents with a characteristic triad of **recurrent abdominal and joint pain, symmetric, palpable purpura** over the buttocks and ankles, and **GI bleeding**.
Epidemiology	Seen more frequently in **males**, usually 2 to 5 years old, especially those with a history of **allergy** or **preceding URIs**.
Management	Treatment is often unnecessary. **Prednisone and analgesics** help ease severe joint and abdominal pain. Improvement is usually seen within 1 month.
Complications	**Intussusception**, progressive **glomerulonephritis**, renal failure, and testicular torsion.
Atlas Links	UCV2 **PED-019A, PED-019B**

HENOCH–SCHÖNLEIN PURPURA

ID/CC A 4-year-old girl is seen for **easy bruising** and a generalized nonpruritic **rash** of 3 days' duration.

HPI She is a healthy child except for a history of easy bruising and frequent nosebleeds that started after a **URI 2 weeks ago**. She is not taking any medications.

PE VS: normal. PE: buccal and conjunctival **mucosal petechiae; [A] generalized small, red, flat subcutaneous macules** that do not blanch on pressure (PETECHIAL RASH), distributed primarily on **pressure points**; no splenomegaly.

Labs CBC/PBS: slight anemia (Hb 10.2); **platelet count decreased**, with giant platelets (MEGATHROMBOCYTES). **PT/PTT normal**; bone marrow shows **normal megakaryocytes** (indicating peripheral bone marrow destruction); **anti-platelet IgG antibodies** present.

Imaging CXR/KUB: normal.

Pathogenesis Thrombocytopenic purpura is an idiopathic condition in which antibodies are formed against one's own platelets (resulting in splenic destruction and thrombocytopenia with bleeding tendency); it generally occurs 2 to 3 weeks after an infection (usually a URI) and is usually associated with a history of nasal, gum, or urinary bleeding. The rash is petechial, and platelets are characteristically low, with prolonged bleeding time. The childhood form is usually acute and self-limited; the adult form is chronic.

Epidemiology Acute, severe thrombocytopenia following a viral URI or exanthem is seen most commonly among children. The chronic

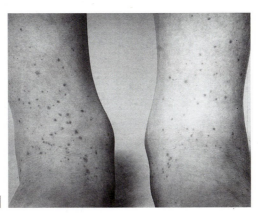

[A]

form is common among adults, particularly women (between 20 and 40 years), who outnumber men by a ratio of 3 to 1.

Management   The disease is **usually self-limited** with resolution of petechiae within 1 to 2 weeks and normalization of platelet count within 6 months. Treat more severe cases (platelets < 20,000) with **steroids, IVIG**, or **Rh (D) immune globulin**. **Splenectomy** should be performed only if the disease is treatment resistant after 12 months. Avoid aspirin and trauma.

Complications   Intracranial bleeding.

Atlas Link   PED-020

ID/CC   A 2-year-old **black** male presents with **painful swelling of the hands and feet** (DACTYLITIS), fever, headache, and a feeling of heaviness in the abdomen (splenomegaly).

HPI   The child has had **recurrent abdominal and joint pain** (due to ischemia). He has also been wetting his bed (ENURESIS) recently. The child's cousin also suffers from a blood disorder.

PE   VS: **fever** (38.3°C). PE: **in pain; pallor** of conjunctiva, skin, and mucous membranes (due to anemia); mild icterus (due to hemolysis); hypoxic spots with neovascularization on retina; throat hyperemic; regular rate and rhythm with no murmurs; lungs clear; **splenomegaly**; skin over metacarpals and metatarsals is warm to touch; **joints tender**.

Labs   CBC/PBS: **[A] sickle-shaped erythrocytes; anemia**; Howell-Jolly bodies and target cells; **reticulocytosis**; leukocytosis; thrombocytosis. LFTs: hyperbilirubinemia (unconjugated); increased LDH. Absent haptoglobin; sickling of RBCs when exposed to sodium metabisulfite (screening); electrophoresis shows **predominantly HbS**, some HbF, and no HbA (ADULT). UA: microscopic hematuria.

Imaging   XR, hands and feet: soft tissue swelling with radiolucent areas (bone necrosis).

Pathogenesis   Sickle cell anemia is an **autosomal-recessive hemoglobinopathy** (HbS) due to a mutation in the gene coding for the β chain of hemoglobin (**glutamic acid substitution for valine at position 6**).

Epidemiology   Incidence is **1 in 400 African Americans** (most common hemoglobinopathy in blacks); 7% of black Americans have the sickle cell trait. **Dactylitis** is the most frequent initial manifestation.

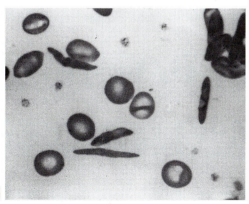

[A]

SICKLE CELL ANEMIA

Onset is at 6 to 12 months, when HbF (which confers protection against sickling) disappears.

Management   Treat crises with **pain control** (avoid meperidine owing to risk of normeperidine accumulation and seizures) and **aggressive hydration**. Transfuse if more anemic than baseline (sickle cell patients are chronically anemic). Treat infections. Laser therapy for retinopathy. Other measures include vaccination against *Haemophilus influenzae* B, hepatitis, and pneumococcus as well as penicillin prophylaxis. Administer hydroxyurea (may increase HbF level). Oxygen, folic acid, exchange transfusion (for stroke prevention, preoperatively, or for priapism), and marrow transplant may be given in severe cases. Prevent crises by avoiding acidosis, hypoxia, hypothermia, dehydration and hyperviscosity states.

Complications   **Autosplenectomy** (due to repeated thrombosis), which increases the risk of bacterial infections by encapsulated organisms (e.g., meningitis, pneumonia, and *Salmonella* **osteomyelitis**), bone infarction with necrosis (RBCs sickling in the sinusoids), anesthetic complications, zinc deficiency, chronic leg ulcers, aseptic necrosis of the femoral head, retinal infarcts, renal papillary necrosis, cerebrovascular infarcts, and acute chest syndrome (pulmonary infarction).

Atlas Links   U̲C̲V̲1̲ H-P2-036, PM-P2-036

ID/CC A 13-year-old girl presents with **prolonged** (> 7 days) **and excessive** (> 50 mL) **menses** that began with menarche 2 weeks ago.

HPI She has a history of **recurrent nosebleeds** (EPISTAXIS), easy bruising, and **prolonged bleeding** from scratches and cuts. Her father also has a bleeding problem.

PE VS: normal. PE: nasal mucosa bleeds excessively with nasal speculum examination; **petechial lesions** seen on arms, legs, and back of chest; bright red blood with clots in vaginal vault.

Labs CBC: anemia; normal platelets. Normal PT; **prolonged bleeding time**; moderately **prolonged aPTT** (intrinsic system); reduced factor VIII by quantitative assay; low von Willebrand factor (vWF); ristocetin cofactor assay shows decreased platelet aggregation.

Imaging CXR/KUB: normal.

Pathogenesis Von Willebrand's disease is most commonly inherited as an **autosomal-dominant** bleeding disorder characterized by **impaired platelet aggregation induced by ristocetin**. Normally, vWF is secreted by endothelial cells and binds platelet surface receptor Gp1b, bridging platelet to subendothelial matrix to form the initial hemostatic plug. Deficient or dysfunctional vWF therefore results in prolonged bleeding time. Since vWF also serves as a plasma carrier for factor VIII, its deficiency is accompanied by reduced factor VIII activity.

Epidemiology The **most common congenital disorder of hemostasis** (more common than hemophilia); seen in both sexes.

Management **Avoid aspirin**, provide reassurance, and **administer factor VIII concentrate. Desmopressin** is used for the treatment of type I (reduced quantity of protein) and for bleeding prophylaxis before surgical procedures (including dental), complemented by tranexamic acid (antifibrinolytic) to prevent bleeding. Desmopressin may not be effective in patients with von Willebrand's disease type II (abnormal quantity of protein) or type III (total absence of protein).

VON WILLEBRAND'S DISEASE

ID/CC	A 7-year-old **boy** is admitted to the hospital for evaluation of a **suspected immune deficiency**.
HPI	During infancy, the child had **atopic dermatitis**. His mother adds that he has had **recurrent skin, ear, and chest infections**. He also has recurrent episodes of **epistaxis**.
PE	VS: normal. PE: **eczematous skin rash** over flexor skin surfaces; **dry, lichenified skin lesions** over face, arms, and extremities; **bilateral otitis media**.
Labs	CBC: anemia; **thrombocytopenia**. Normal levels of IgG; **high levels of IgE and IgA; reduced levels of IgM**; anergic to bacterial and fungal antigens; **nitroblue tetrazolium test normal**.
Imaging	CXR: normal.
Pathogenesis	Wiskott–Aldrich syndrome is a disorder of both B and T cell immunity and is characterized by **eczema, thrombocytopenia, and increased susceptibility to infection** (mainly encapsulated organisms). The gene for Wiskott–Aldrich syndrome has been mapped to the X chromosome. The syndrome is associated with secondary malignancies, especially non-Hodgkin's lymphoma. Survival to adulthood is rare given increased susceptibility to infection, bleeding, and malignancy.
Epidemiology	An **X-linked recessive** disease seen predominantly in males.
Management	Requires **bone marrow transplantation** after administering irradiation or busulfan and antilymphocyte serum to destroy residual lymphocytes. Patients have subsequently shown normal immune and platelet function.
Complications	Infection and malignancy.

ID/CC	A **1-year-old** boy presents with **respiratory distress, coughing** (dry and hacking; sometimes paroxysmal), and **wheezing**.
HPI	Immunizations are up to date. Others in his day-care center have had similar symptoms. The boy had a runny nose 2 days ago.
PE	VS: **tachycardia; marked tachypnea; low-grade fever**. PE: in acute distress; **dyspnea** noted (nasal flaring, intercostal retraction, and use of accessory muscles of respiration); no cyanosis (vs. pertussis and epiglottitis); no conjunctivitis (vs. chlamydial pneumonia); no drooling (vs. epiglottitis); **audible expiratory wheezes**; no inspiratory stridor (vs. croup); **rales, crackles, and rhonchi** heard on auscultation.
Labs	CBC: leukocytosis with **lymphocytosis**. ABGs: **hypoxemia**. Sputum culture reveals **normal flora**; pertussis culture negative; **viral culture RSV positive** (gold standard); nasopharyngeal washings (ELISA or immunofluorescence) RSV positive.
Imaging	CXR: **hyperinflation** with air trapping, flattened diaphragms, increased bronchovascular markings, peribronchial cuffing, segmental **atelectasis**, and **interstitial infiltrates**.
Pathogenesis	Bronchiolitis is a lower respiratory tract infection of viral origin, usually **RSV**, in which epithelial necrosis, increased mucus, and edema lead to obstruction and atelectasis. At increased risk are immune-compromised patients, premature infants, and those with congenital heart diseases or underlying pulmonary disease.
Epidemiology	Usually **symptomatic in children 6 to 12 months** of age; less symptomatic in children older than 2 years. Occurs in yearly epidemics, primarily in **winter** and **spring**.
Management	Management is primarily **supportive**: nutrition (IV or NG tube), humidified oxygen, nebulized β_2-agonists, and ventilatory support. Ribavirin is given in severe cases. Amantadine should be given in the presence of influenza virus; prophylactic monoclonal antibody to RSV can be given in the presence of pulmonary disease, epidemics, or prematurity. Most patients recover in approximately four days.
Complications	Bacterial superinfection (otitis media, bronchitis, bronchopneumonia), cyanosis, apneic spells, respiratory insufficiency, fatigue, dehydration (from poor feeding), and chronic hyperreactive airways.

ACUTE BRONCHIOLITIS

ID/CC A 7-year-old boy presents with **fever, pain and swelling of the elbows and knees**, and a **skin rash** on his trunk and arms of 2 days' duration.

HPI The patient is otherwise healthy with no relevant past medical history. Two weeks ago, he suffered from a **sore throat**, high **fever**, and generalized weakness. He has no history of tick bites.

PE VS: **fever** (38.5°C); tachycardia; normal BP. PE: **confluent, serpiginous, nonpruritic erythematous rash** over trunk and proximal extremities (ERYTHEMA MARGINATUM); **subcutaneous nodules** (which are painless, firm, and 3 to 4 mm in diameter) on extensor tendons of MCP joints and elbow as well as on posterior scalp; swollen, red knee and elbow joints (POLYARTHRITIS); pedal edema; elevated JVP; high-frequency apical systolic murmur with radiation to axilla (mitral insufficiency due to carditis); bilateral fine inspiratory rales; mild tender hepatomegaly.

Labs CBC: **leukocytosis** (14,900) with **neutrophilia** (85%). **Increased ASO** titer and anti-DNase (evidence of preceding streptococcal infection); **elevated ESR** (useful for following disease activity; remains elevated for months); elevated C-reactive protein (CRP); culture of throat swab grows *Streptococcus pyogenes*; blood culture negative. ECG: changing P-wave contour and **prolonged PR interval with small QRS complexes** (due to ventricular dilatation and small pericardial effusion).

Imaging CXR: **cardiomegaly**; increased pulmonary vascular markings; very small left pleural effusion. Echo: vegetations over the mitral valve with regurgitation.

Pathogenesis Rheumatic fever is a sequela of infection with **group A β-hemolytic streptococci** that causes autoimmune heart damage; it typically occurs 2 weeks after streptococcal pharyngitis (unlike glomerulonephritis, carditis does not follow skin infections). **Jones' major criteria** for the diagnosis of rheumatic fever include **pancarditis** (clinical or radiologic evidence of myocarditis, endocarditis, and pericarditis), **polyarthritis** (typically migratory arthritis involving large joints), **Sydenham's chorea** (more frequent in females; involuntary purposeful movements of voluntary muscles), **subcutaneous nodules**, and **erythema marginatum** (migratory pink macular rash seen on the trunk and proximal extremities). **Minor criteria** include **fever, arthralgia, previous rheumatic fever, elevated ESR, elevated CRP**, and **prolonged PR interval**.

The presence of **two major or one major and two minor** criteria plus evidence of a **recent strep infection** (elevated ASO titers, positive throat culture for *S. pyogenes*) is used to diagnose acute rheumatic fever.

Epidemiology The leading cause of acquired heart disease in children, it usually occurs between the ages of 5 and 15.

Management Treat infection. Give aspirin, steroids (indicated for severe carditis), bed rest. Administer digoxin and diuretics in the presence of CHF and diazepam for chorea. ESR takes months to return to normal. Prophylaxis every month with benzathine penicillin to prevent recurrences (more common in younger children and in those who had carditis; usually appears in the first few years after rheumatic fever).

Complications Arrhythmias, pericardial effusion, pneumonitis, and valvular heart defects (more commonly affects the mitral valve).

Atlas Link 🅤🅒🅥🅘 M-M1-052

MINICASE 323: CMV—CONGENITAL

The most common viral infection transmitted from mother to fetus
- more likely to be transmitted when the mother is newly infected during pregnancy
- presents with floppiness, lethargy, poor feeding, small size for gestational age, hepatosplenomegaly, jaundice, petechiae, seizures, and chorioretinitis
- anemia, thrombocytopenia, elevated LFTs, CMV IgM, urine positive for CMV culture, and early antigen (between 2 days and 1 week of age)
- x-ray of the skull shows microcephaly and CT of the head shows intracerebral calcifications
- treat infant with acyclovir
- complications include severe neurologic, intellectual, visual, and auditory impairment

---

ACUTE RHEUMATIC FEVER

ID/CC	A 10-month-old infant presents with complaints of **severe, intractable, chronic diarrhea** and **failure to thrive**.
HPI	The father reveals that the **mother died of AIDS** shortly after delivery.
PE	VS: mild fever; tachycardia; tachypnea. PE: emaciated and grossly malnourished; oral **thrush**; axillary, cervical, and inguinal **lymphadenopathy; hepatosplenomegaly**.
Labs	**CD4 T-cell count depressed; ELISA** and **Western blot** for HIV-1 **positive** (could be due to maternal antibodies but strongly supports the diagnosis in the presence of symptoms); **PCR viral RNA positive** (confirming HIV infection).
Imaging	CXR: normal.
Pathogenesis	Transmission of HIV-1 from mother to infant most commonly occurs **during delivery** through contact with contaminated blood or secretions. **Transplacental** passage of the virus and postnatal infection through **breast feeding** also occur. Increased risk of infection in the neonate is associated with advanced disease in the mother (**p24 antigenemia**, high level of **HIV-1 RNA in plasma**, and **low CD4+** cell counts).
Epidemiology	Transmission of HIV-1 from mother to infant varies from 13% to 45% in cohort studies conducted in Europe and Africa, respectively, with an average of approximately 25%.
Management	**Zidovudine** (AZT) administered during the **second** and **third trimesters, intrapartum,** and during **the first 6 weeks of life** reduces transmission. Antiretroviral therapy is started when immune suppression or HIV-related symptoms are demonstrated. Administer *Pneumocystis carinii* pneumonia prophylaxis and antimicrobials for specific infections. Pregnancy should be discouraged in female carriers. Children with AIDS should not be given oral polio vaccine, BCG, or varicella. MMR may be given if the child is not overtly immunosuppressed. DTP, hepatitis B, and inactivated polio vaccine can be administered. HIV-positive mothers **should not breast feed** their babies.

ID/CC A 4-month-old infant is seen for **difficulty breast feeding**.

HPI The mother also noticed that the child has been **constipated** for the past few days. The infant has **regularly been given honey** by his grandmother.

PE VS: tachycardia; tachypnea; normal BP. PE: **hypotonic**; breathing appears shallow and labored (**diaphragm weakness**); poor sucking and rooting reflex; weight and height normal for age; no hepatosplenomegaly; **ptosis; pupils dilated** and **sluggishly reacting to light**.

Labs EMG: characteristic pattern of **brief, small, abundant motor-unit action potentials** noted. Normal nerve conduction; stool culture yields *Clostridium botulinum* growth, and toxin detected in feces; *C. botulinum* toxin present in blood. LP: **CSF normal**.

Pathogenesis Botulism in infants is thought to be caused by **colonization** of the intestine and subsequent release of toxin by *C. botulinum,* with later **absorption of the toxin. Honey** has been implicated in at least one-third of cases.

Epidemiology Infant botulism has been reported worldwide. Most cases occur in California, where spores are present in soil and on many vegetables.

Management **Ventilatory** and **nutritional support** are the mainstays of treatment. A human-derived antitoxin is available for infants. Avoid consumption of honey in children younger than 1 year of age. Avoid aminoglycosides (potentiate effect of toxin at neuromuscular junction).

BOTULISM—INFANT

ID/CC	A 9-month-old girl is seen after the development of a **brassy, barking cough**.
HPI	The patient is otherwise healthy and is up to date with her vaccinations. She has also been suffering from a **URI** of 6 days' duration, which is characterized by fever, malaise, rhinorrhea, and a runny nose.
PE	VS: low-grade fever (38.2°C). PE: restless and in **respiratory distress** with suprasternal and intercostal retractions; intermittent **inspiratory stridor; hoarse, barking cough**; diminished breath sounds bilaterally and scattered rales.
Labs	**CBC: normal**.
Imaging	XR, neck: on AP view, **steeple sign** (subglottic narrowing, vs. "thumbprint sign" on lateral view in epiglottitis).
Pathogenesis	Croup is caused primarily by the **parainfluenza virus**. Other offenders include influenza virus, adenovirus, and RSV (although the latter typically produces bronchiolitis).
Epidemiology	Most commonly occurs in patients between the ages of 6 months and 6 years, with a male predominance. Seen more frequently in **fall** and **winter** (during change from warm to cold weather).
Management	Mild cases can be **managed supportively** on an outpatient basis. **Mist therapy**, oxygen, **racemic epinephrine**, acetaminophen, and corticosteroids (if severe) may be useful. Hospitalize if there is stridor at rest.
Complications	Respiratory failure, dehydration due to inability to feed, and pneumonia.

ID/CC	An 8-year-old boy presents with **fever** and chills for 3 days associated with **fatigue, joint pain**, sore throat, and an **extensive skin rash on his left leg**.
HPI	The patient is a native of **Wisconsin** who attended a **summer camp** 7 days ago (incubation 3 to 30 days). On directed questioning, he recalls having noticed a **tick** on his leg while hiking in the forest.
PE	VS: fever (38°C). PE: neurologic exam normal; rash is **nonpruritic**, started as a red spot (erythematous macule) at site of tick bite, and continued to expand in a **ringlike manner with an active border and central clearing**, yielding a **target appearance** (ERYTHEMA CHRONICUM MIGRANS).
Labs	CBC: no anemia or leukocytosis. Elevated ESR; **elevated IgM** for *Borrelia burgdorferi* initially (window period of 2 weeks); **elevated IgG** later (6 weeks); false positives in other spirochete infections, collagen vascular diseases, leptospirosis, and mononucleosis; diagnosis **confirmed by Western blot**; positive blood culture. LP: lymphocytosis; mildly elevated protein; normal glucose.
Pathogenesis	Lyme disease is caused by *__Borrelia burgdorferi__* (a spirochete), which is transmitted by the tick *Ixodes scapularis*. Lyme disease initially presents with a diagnostic rash > 5 cm surrounding the area of the tick bite, whose center may desquamate, ulcerate, or necrose, together with satellite lesions. **Stage I** is characterized by **erythema chronicum migrans**, severe headache, fever, chills, and malaise (atypical cases may resolve spontaneously). **Stage II** occurs weeks afterward and presents with **CNS symptoms** (transverse myelitis, meningoencephalitis, mononeuritis multiplex, dysesthesias, CN palsy, chorea) and **cardiac abnormalities** (conduction disturbances, myocarditis, arrhythmias). **Stage III** occurs weeks to months after initial infection and presents as recurrent, **migratory arthritis**, mainly in the large joints, **synovitis** (silver stain for spirochetes positive, synovial fluid *Borrelia* DNA positive by PCR), and atrophic macules on the fingers and toes (ACRODERMATITIS CHRONICUM ATROPHICANS). The arthritis may be associated with HLA-DR4.
Epidemiology	The **most common vector-borne disease** in the United States, its incidence is increasing; found in the coastal Northeast, California, and the Midwest (clustered around woodlands). It is more common in the summer and early fall. The **tick bite** is usually

painless (24-hour tick attachment is needed for transmission). Reservoir includes deer, mice, and raccoons.

Management   Pediatric disease can be managed with **amoxicillin** (avoid tetracycline). Prevention consists of avoidance of wooded areas, clothing protection, repellent, and, if noted, prompt tick removal. Consider post-tick-bite antibiotic prophylaxis if endemic. A vaccine is now available.

Complications   Dissemination, subacute encephalopathy, leukoencephalitis, cardiac conduction defects, polyneuritis, and musculoskeletal disorders. Complications are rare in children.

MINICASE 324: DIPHTHERIA

An acute contagious disease caused by toxigenic strains of *Corynebacterium diphtheriae* in unvaccinated patients
- presents in children with sore throat, malaise, fever, cervical adenopathy, and a whitish-gray adherent membrane over the tonsils and pharynx
- Albert's stain of throat culture shows metachromatic granules in bacilli arranged in "Chinese character" pattern, growth seen on Löffler's/tellurite blood agar
- treat with supportive care (bed rest, oxygenation, endotracheal intubation or tracheostomy as indicated), antitoxin, and antibiotics (penicillin or erythromycin until two cultures are negative)
- complications include CHF and conduction abnormalities (secondary to toxigenic myocarditis), dysphagia (due to bulbar paralysis), and peripheral nerve palsies

Atlas Links: UCV2 MC-324   UCV1 M-M1-082

MINICASE 325: MUMPS

Infection caused by the paramyxovirus, most commonly involving the parotid gland
- the incidence of mumps has decreased dramatically since the advent of the mumps vaccine
- presents with a prodrome of malaise, fever, chills, and a sore throat, followed by swelling in one or both parotid glands
- although diagnosis is usually clinical, CBC may show leukopenia, and serum amylase may be elevated
- treat complications supportively including orchitis, oophoritis, pancreatitis, and encephalitis

ID/CC   A **16-month-old** girl presents to the emergency room with failure to thrive, fever, cough, and a **rash of 1 week's duration**.

HPI   Her parents report that the child has become increasingly irritable and fatigued and has demonstrated increasingly poor oral intake over the past week. They add that she has also had a persistent, nonproductive **cough**, a runny nose (**coryza**), sneezing, and **conjunctivitis**. Three days ago the parents noted a red **rash that appeared first on the face** and behind the ears and then **"moved" down to the trunk and palms**. The child's fever was as high as 40°C but is now decreasing.

PE   VS: fever (39.1°C); tachycardia (HR 130); tachypnea (RR 24). PE: small, poorly nourished, and in moderate distress; erythematous, nonpruritic, **maculopapular rash** noted along length of trunk and bilateral palms and soles with some confluence of lesions; small, 1- to 2-mm **bluish-white spots** (KOPLIK'S SPOTS) noted on inflamed, erythematous oral mucous membranes and buccal mucosa; mild **oropharyngeal edema** with yellow exudate on tonsils; moderate cervical lymphadenopathy bilaterally; lungs clear.

Labs   CBC: WBC count 1,800. UA: 2+ protein on urine dipstick.

Imaging   CXR: normal (may often be abnormal owing to frequent secondary bacterial pneumonias).

Pathogenesis   The measles virus invades the respiratory epithelium and spreads via blood to the skin, respiratory tract, GI tract, and reticuloendothelial system, where it infects all WBC types. Virions are generally transmitted by respiratory secretions, predominantly through aerosol exposure but also through direct contact; patients are contagious from 1 to 2 days before the onset of symptoms until 4 days after the rash appears. The mean interval from infection to onset of symptoms is approximately 10 days; the time to onset of rash is approximately 14 days.

Epidemiology   Measles has a worldwide distribution, and humans are the only natural hosts. A recent resurgence of cases has been noted during the 1990s due to failure to immunize infants and young children in the inner cities. However, the standard vaccination protocol has resulted in the reporting of < 300 cases per year to the CDC. The majority of cases continue to be found in preschool children, with the highest mortality found in children younger than 2 years and among adults. Worldwide pediatric mortality continues to be > 1 million each year.

Management   **Primary prevention** is central to disease control. The current recommendation suggests that the first **vaccination** be given between the ages of 12 and 15 months and the second at 4 to 6 years (prior to entry into school). Preschool children younger than 1 year may be given their initial vaccination as early as 6 months old in the presence of outbreaks. Susceptible individuals exposed to the measles virus can be protected if they are given the live virus vaccine within 72 hours of exposure or gamma globulin within 6 days of exposure. The vaccine should not be used in pregnant women or immune-compromised individuals. Patients with measles should be **isolated** for 1 week following the development of the rash. Treatment is supportive. Antibiotics, bed rest, adequate fluid and vitamin A supplementation are recommended.

Complications   The mortality rate of this condition is 1 in 1,000 in the United States; death is primarily related to CNS encephalitis and bacterial pneumonias. Respiratory complications include viral bronchopneumonia or bronchiolitis (1% to 7%); CNS complications are common and include acute encephalitis (fever, headache, drowsiness, coma, and seizures), which occurs in 1 in 1,000 patients, has an onset 3 to 7 days after the rash, and carries a high mortality rate (10% to 20%). **Subacute sclerosing panencephalitis** is an extremely rare complication (1 in 100,000) involving a delayed neurodegenerative process; usually seen following infection in males younger than 2 years old. This entity manifests as progressive dementia years after the initial infection. Secondary bacterial infections such as otitis media (the most frequent complication) and cervical adenitis are common; GI complications such as gastroenteritis, hepatitis, appendicitis, ileocolitis, and mesenteric adenitis are also seen.

Atlas Links   🆄🅲🆅2 **PED-030A, PED-030B**

MINICASE 326: RUBELLA—CONGENITAL

Can be transmitted to the fetus in utero by maternal infection in early pregnancy
- classically presents with cataracts, heart disease, and deafness along with low birth weight, hepatosplenomegaly, and mental retardation
- labs reveal thrombocytopenia and leukopenia, rubella virus isolated from urine and saliva, markedly increased IgM-specific antibody for rubella
- treatment is supportive
- preventable by vaccination with MMR prior to pregnancy

ID/CC A 9-year-old Boy Scout presents with **sudden-onset fever, chills, headache, lethargy**, and **abdominal pain** of 4 days' duration.

HPI Earlier today he developed a **rash that began on his wrists and ankles** and spread to the trunk. He is a healthy boy with no relevant past medical history who went **camping in North Carolina** 10 days ago. Directed questioning reveals that he suffered a **tick bite** on his lower leg.

PE VS: **fever** (39.1°C); tachycardia (HR 129); normal BP. PE: slight **icterus**; face flushed and **conjunctiva injected**; generalized non-tender rash of small, bright red confluent macules (early) and petechiae (later), some of them hemorrhagic and necrotic, on soles, palms, wrists, ankles, arms, trunk, and abdomen (due to vasculitis); mild hepatosplenomegaly.

Labs CBC: slight **leukopenia** (5,000); thrombocytopenia. Lytes: hyponatremia. UA: proteinuria. Skin biopsy (positive early) and serologic immunofluorescence positive for *Rickettsia rickettsii*; Weil-Felix positive.

Pathogenesis Rocky Mountain spotted fever is caused by *Rickettsia rickettsii* and is transmitted by *Dermacentor andersoni* tick bite (hosts are dogs and rodents); it is characterized by a **typical triad** of **history of tick exposure, fever**, and **generalized centripetal rash**. The rash **characteristically involves the palms and soles**. At times, however, the disease appears without a rash.

Epidemiology Commonly occurs in the spring and summer; the incubation period is usually 2 to 14 days. More prevalent on the **East Coast** (primarily in Virginia and North Carolina) and in the Southeast. The overall mortality rate is significantly reduced with treatment.

Management Treat dehydration and electrolyte imbalance. Give **chloramphenicol** for at least 1 week for children younger than 8 years. **Doxycycline** may be given to older children.

Complications Myocarditis, pneumonitis, gangrene of digits, acute renal failure, residual convulsions, DIC, ARDS, and cerebral edema.

ID/CC	A 6-year-old boy presents with an **inability to hear**.
HPI	The child's mother is an immigrant who received no **prenatal care**. At birth he appeared normal. The mother states that the child also appears **developmentally delayed**, with speech problems. He has exhibited photophobia and increased lacrimation.
PE	VS: normal. PE: **saddlenose** and **poorly developed maxilla; centrally notched** (due to defectively formed enamel), **widely spaced, small, peg-shaped upper incisors** (HUTCHINSON'S TEETH); thickening of anterior tibial area (**saber shins**); optic atrophy and exudative vascularization of the cornea.
Labs	**Positive RPR** and FTA-ABS.
Imaging	XR, long bones: osseous abnormalities include luetic metaphysitis, diaphysitis, and periostitis; symmetric destruction of the medial portion of the proximal tibial metaphyses (WIMBERGER'S SIGN) is pathognomonic; diffuse anterior thickening of the upper half of the tibial cortex (SABER TIBIA).
Pathogenesis	Congenital syphilis is caused by *Treponema pallidum*, a spirochete that may cross the placenta at any stage of pregnancy. Adequate treatment prior to gestational week 18 generally prevents fetal sequelae. Prior to this time, the fetal immune system is incompetent, suggesting that the damage results from the fetal immune response to *T. pallidum* rather than from direct toxicity. The most characteristic **triad** of late congenital syphilis consists of **interstitial keratitis, Hutchinson's teeth**, and **eighth nerve deafness**. Since maternal-fetal transmission is rare before the fifth month, syphilis is an uncommon cause of abortion.
Epidemiology	One in 10,000 live newborn infants is infected. With untreated primary maternal syphilis, the rate of transmission is 75% to 90%. With maternal infection of 2 years or more, the rate of transmission is 35%.
Management	Penicillin G is the only recommended therapy. **Empiric treatment** is indicated in neonates who may not have follow-up and whose status is equivocal. All women should receive **screening** at their first prenatal visit and at delivery; women at high risk should receive repeat screenings.
Complications	Stillbirth, prematurity, and mental retardation.

ID/CC	A 10-day-old male infant presents with **marked muscle rigidity and spasm**.
HPI	The mother did not receive any prenatal care, and the child was delivered at home. The child has **not received any immunizations**.
PE	VS: tachycardia; tachypnea. PE: extremely ill-looking with **generalized rigidity** and **opisthotonos; spasm worsens** with agitation; jaw muscle rigidity (TRISMUS).
Labs	CBC/Lytes/ABGs: normal. Culture of **umbilical stump** yields *Clostridium tetani*.
Pathogenesis	Tetanus is caused by *Clostridium tetani*, a **gram-positive, motile, nonencapsulated, anaerobic, spore-bearing bacillus** that produces a **powerful neurotoxin** (tetanospasmin). The toxin acts principally on **the spinal cord** (inhibits the release of glycine, an inhibitory neurotransmitter). The characteristic clinical features are determined by the relative strengths of the opposing muscles. For example, the greater strength of the masseter over the opposing digastricus and mylohyoid results in **trismus**. The combination of flexion of the upper extremities and extension of the lower extremities is termed **opisthotonos**.
Epidemiology	The cause of numerous infant deaths in developing countries, most attributable to the lack of tetanus immunization and the use of contaminated material to cut the umbilical cord.
Management	Provide ventilatory assistance; maintain nutrition and fluid and electrolyte balance; give **IM tetanus** IgG. Give **penicillin G**; control tetanic spasms with diazepam. **Debride devitalized tissue** where *C. tetani* is growing. **Immunize pregnant women** with tetanus toxoid and maintain proper asepsis during delivery.
Complications	Notable complications include aspiration pneumonia, **respiratory failure**, rhabdomyolysis (from sustained seizure activity), and autonomic nervous system dysfunction (cardiac arrhythmias, unstable BP, temperature instability, and epileptic seizures).

ID/CC	A **newborn baby** is seen for an **extensive maculopapular rash** and **fever**.
HPI	His mother received no prenatal care and lives alone with a **pet cat**. She did not report any rashes or illnesses during pregnancy.
PE	VS: tachycardia; moderate tachypnea; fever. PE: **small for gestational age**; microcephalic with **extensive maculopapular rash** (spares soles, palms, and scalp); **jaundice; chorioretinitis** with yellow-white, fluffy exudates clustered in posterior pole; **hepatosplenomegaly**.
Labs	CBC: thrombocytopenia. IFA for **IgM antibodies positive**; ELISA for IgM positive; **ToRCH test** on maternal serum (To = *Toxoplasma*, R = rubella, C = CMV, H = herpes zoster) also positive for *Toxoplasma* **infection**; serologic tests for syphilis, CMV, HIV, and rubella negative in neonate.
Imaging	XR, skull: **calcifications**. CT, head: **diffuse cerebral calcification** (vs. periventricular calcification seen in CMV inclusion disease).
Pathogenesis	*Toxoplasma gondii,* **an obligate intracellular protozoan** parasite, is the causative agent in toxoplasmosis. Infection via the oral route is caused by the ingestion of *T. gondii* cysts in undercooked food or by the ingestion of *T. gondii* oocysts, which are found in **cat feces**. If the **initial infection occurs during pregnancy**, parasitemia can cause **transplacental infection** of the fetus. Mothers with **chronic or latent toxoplasmosis** acquired before pregnancy **do not transmit** the infection to their children.
Epidemiology	Most infants with congenital toxoplasmosis will show clinical evidence of infection by adolescence if not treated at birth.
Management	**Pyrimethamine and sulfadiazine** used in combination for afflicted infants; folinic acid to prevent bone marrow suppression. Spiramycin should be started immediately for pregnant women. **Therapeutic abortion** might be considered if the infection is acquired early in pregnancy. Prevention is key and involves **avoidance** by minimizing contact with **cat feces** (not changing the cat litter) and not eating **undercooked meat**.

ID/CC	An 8-year-old girl presents with **fever** of 5 days' duration and an **itchy skin rash** that **started on her face and trunk** and **spread to her extremities**.
HPI	Lesions have appeared in **successive crops**. Four classmates recently missed school due to similar symptoms.
PE	VS: **fever** (39.1°C); tachycardia. PE: well hydrated and nourished; lesions consist of **macules** (earliest), **papules, vesicles, pustules, and scabs, all present simultaneously** and appearing predominantly over trunk, face, and scalp; lungs clear; no hepatosplenomegaly; neurologic exam normal.
Labs	CBC: **leukopenia** (4,500). **Multinucleated giant cells** on Tzanck smears of vesicle base scraping; specific complement fixation and fluorescent antibody test positive.
Imaging	CXR: no evidence of pneumonitis (a potential complication).
Pathogenesis	Varicella is also known as **chickenpox**; it is caused by the **varicella-zoster virus** (a DNA herpesvirus). Spread by **direct contact** and **respiratory droplets**. Transmissible from 24–48 hours before the rash appears until lesions have crusted over.
Epidemiology	A **highly contagious** infection that occurs in epidemics; more common in **late winter** and **early spring**.
Management	Treat with **oral antihistamines** (avoid topical), **acetaminophen** (avoid aspirin due to risk of Reye's syndrome), oatmeal soap, and calamine lotion; clip fingernails (to prevent excoriation). Give prophylactic, postexposure (from 5 days before delivery to 2 days after) **varicella-zoster immune globulin** to newborns, immune-compromised patients, pregnant mothers, and adults older than 25 years old. **Acyclovir** can be given to immune-compromised patients and infants as well as in severe cases. Prevent through use of **live attenuated vaccine**.
Complications	Complications include **skin infection** (most common), arthritis, myocarditis, thrombocytopenia (skin, mucous membranes, and vesicle hemorrhages), scarlet fever (strep infection), encephalitis (varicella cerebellitis), **pneumonitis** (in older patients, carries risk of ARDS), nephrotic syndrome, HUS, **Reye's syndrome** (with ASA), **herpes zoster** (SHINGLES; reactivation of dormant virus in nerves), and visceral involvement in immune-compromised patients (transplant patients, cancer patients undergoing

VARICELLA ZOSTER (CHICKENPOX)

chemotherapy, those on steroids, patients with HIV). In pregnant patients, complications can include low birth weight, deafness, cataracts, and chorioretinitis in the fetus.

Atlas Links   ⬛UCV2⬛ **PED-035**   ⬛UCV1⬛ M-M2-074

MINICASE 327: WHOOPING COUGH

Caused by a toxin produced by *Bordetella pertussis*
- presents in three stages: a catarrhal stage with sneezing and nocturnal cough, a paroxysmal stage with frequent productive "whooping cough" with vomiting, and a slow convalescent stage
- nasal swab culture reveals organism, labs show marked lymphocytosis
- treat with oxygen as needed
- place the patient in strict respiratory isolation, give erythromycin to decrease the duration of the carrier state

---

VARICELLA ZOSTER (CHICKENPOX)

ID/CC	A 2-year-old **boy** presents with fever, cough, and irritability.
HPI	He contracted his first respiratory tract infection at approximately 9 months of age and has had numerous **bacterial infections** since then.
PE	VS: fever (39°C); tachypnea (RR 40); tachycardia (HR 130). PE: grunting respirations; **tonsils absent on inspection**; flaring of alae nasi; intercostal retractions; use of accessory muscles of respiration; **crackles at right base** (pneumonia).
Labs	CBC: elevated WBC (15,000); normal lymphocyte counts. Sputum Gram stain reveals gram-positive cocci in chains; **markedly depressed IgA, IgG, IgE, and IgM levels; total immunoglobulin levels < 100 mg/dL; lymph node biopsy reveals absence of germinal centers**.
Imaging	CXR: focal right lower lobe infiltrate.
Pathogenesis	Bruton's agammaglobulinemia is also known as **X-linked agammaglobulinemia**. It is caused by a **defect in a nonreceptor tyrosine kinase** involved in signal transduction; the defect leads to a developmental block and arrest at the pre-B-cell level. A small number of B cells progress to maturation and exist in the periphery as plasma cells; however, this occurs at a relatively low frequency. As a result, patients are **highly susceptible to bacterial infections**, particularly within the respiratory tract and by encapsulated organisms.
Epidemiology	Develops in **boys**, with the first sequelae of the disease appearing late in the first year of life following the disappearance of maternal immunoglobulins. Females may serve as carriers but are unaffected.
Management	Administer **monthly IV immunoglobulin**, which replenishes IgG but not IgA. Doses should be titrated to maintain a trough IgG level in excess of 400 mg/dL.
Complications	Patients may develop chronic meningoencephalitis secondary to echovirus infection, dermatomyositis, arthritis similar to rheumatoid arthritis, and diarrhea secondary to *Giardia lamblia*.

IMMUNOLOGY

BRUTON'S AGAMMAGLOBULINEMIA

ID/CC An 8-month-old boy is seen for **gradual-onset breathing difficulties** (due to *Pneumocystis carinii* pneumonia).

HPI The child also has a low-grade **fever**, a nonproductive **cough**, and **chronic diarrhea**. His mother states that he also has a history of **multiple candidal skin infections**.

PE VS: **fever; tachypnea**; tachycardia; normal BP. PE: **cachectic**; cyanosis and dyspnea noted; **alopecia** (almost universal feature) with abundant **seborrhea** on scalp and forehead; scattered rales in lungs.

Labs CBC: **marked lymphopenia**; neutropenia; **anemia** (of chronic disease); increased platelets (THROMBOCYTOSIS). Anergic response to PPD; hypogammaglobulinemia; increased lymphocyte AMP; **low adenosine deaminase** (ADA) **activity in RBCs**. ABGs: hypoxemia.

Imaging CXR: **no thymic shadow** (THYMIC APLASIA). **[A]** CXR: patchy infiltrates bilaterally (atypical pneumonia).

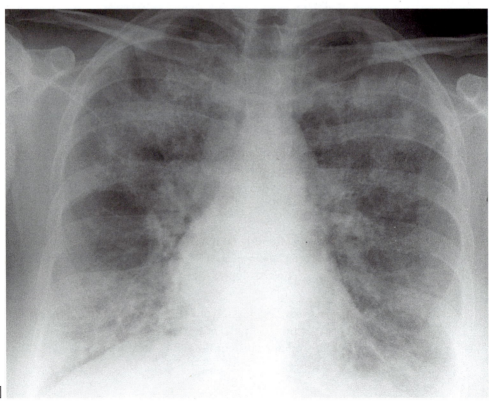

[A]

Pathogenesis	Severe combined immunodeficiency is a heterogeneous group of disorders caused by **defective lymphocyte development**. Defective B-lymphocyte development results in **humoral immune deficiency (hypogammaglobulinemia)**; defective T-lymphocyte development results in **cellular immune deficiency** (absent delayed-type hypersensitivity). **ADA deficiency** is a variant that accounts for 20% of cases. Most patients present with *Pneumocystis* pneumonia.
Epidemiology	A relatively rare immune deficiency; most patients die within the first year of life due to sepsis.
Management	**Bone marrow transplant** offers the best chance of cure. Start TMP-SMX for *Pneumocystis* **prophylaxis; IgG replacement** when the diagnosis is known. Give antibiotics for infection; avoid blood transfusions (graft-versus-host disease).

MINICASE 328: CHRONIC GRANULOMATOUS DISEASE

An X-linked disorder due to a deficiency of NADPH oxidase in neutrophils
• presents with recurrent infections with *Staphylococcus*, *Serratia* and fungi
• neutrophilic leukocytosis, absence of respiratory burst, and a negative NBT
• treat infections appropriately, consider chronic Bactrim prophylaxis

MINICASE 329: DIGEORGE'S SYNDROME

Due to an embryologic defect characterized by lack of development of the third and fourth pharyngeal pouches, leading to a lack of thymus and parathyroid glands as well as to cardiac defects
• presents with increased muscle tone, oral thrush, midfacial hypoplasia, tetany, truncus arteriosus, and recurrent URIs
• labs reveal hypocalcemia, markedly low T-cell count, CXR shows absence of thymic shadow
• treat with supportive care (antibiotics for opportunistic infections, calcium replacement for hypocalcemic tetany, transfusion of irradiated blood products), transplant of an immature fetal thymus

MINICASE 330: HEREDITARY ANGIOEDEMA

An autosomal-dominant deficiency of C1 esterase inhibitor
- presents with episodic, diffuse soft tissue swelling, recurrent attacks of GI colic, and laryngeal edema
- decreased C4 and C2 due to excessive complement activation
- treat with danazol to stimulate C1 esterase inhibitor production from functional allele
- complications can include laryngeal edema and respiratory failure

MINICASE: 330

ID/CC A newborn infant with a **low Apgar** score is evaluated.

HPI The neonate has been **cyanotic since birth**, and his color does not improve when he cries (unlike choanal atresia). The mother did not undergo any prenatal ultrasound screening for birth defects.

PE Full-term male neonate with cyanosis; **breath sounds absent on left side; heart sounds shifted** toward right; occasional **peristaltic movements heard over left side of chest; abdomen is scaphoid.**

Labs ABGs: hypoxemia.

Imaging CXR: **loops of intestine herniating through the diaphragmatic defect** into the left side of the chest with the heart shifted toward the right. **[A]** CXR: another case demonstrates a right diaphragmatic defect and bowel loops in the right thorax (1), displacing the esophagus (NG tube) (2) to the left. US, fetal: bowel loops in chest with incomplete diaphragm.

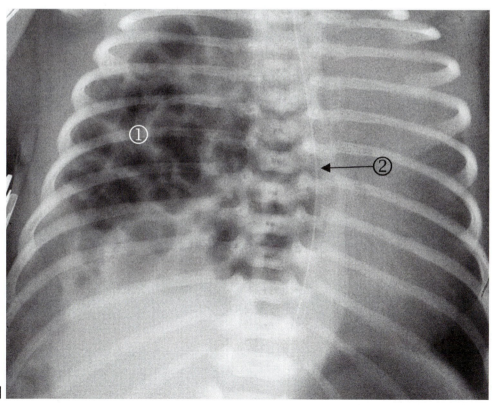

[A]

38   CONGENITAL DIAPHRAGMATIC HERNIA

Pathogenesis	There are two types of congenital diaphragmatic hernia; most commonly, a posterolateral defect in the diaphragm (**Bochdalek hernia**) is involved, but approximately 5% of cases are due to a retrosternal defect (**Morgagni hernia**). These defects allow abdominal viscera to enter the thorax and compromise lung development. Embryologically, the diaphragm is derived from the septum transversum, pleuroperitoneal folds, dorsal esophageal mesentery, and body wall.
Epidemiology	**Ninety percent** of diaphragmatic hernias occur on the **left side**.
Management	**Ventilatory support** and **surgical repair** are required. Restrictive lung disease, reactive lung disease, neurologic abnormalities, pectus excavatum, scoliosis, and recurrent herniation may result. High-frequency ventilation or extracorporeal membrane oxygenation (ECMO) may be needed to treat pulmonary hypertension.
Complications	Pulmonary hypertension due to prolonged intubation; infections.

MINICASE 331: MECONIUM ASPIRATION

The most common cause of neonatal respiratory distress in full-term infants
- due to bronchial obstruction by meconium
- presents with acute cyanosis at birth
- CXR shows consolidation, infiltrates, and atelectasis
- treat with aggressive suctioning, intubation if necessary, high-flow oxygen

---

MINICASE 332: MECONIUM ILEUS

Intestinal obstruction in the neonatal period due to accumulation of viscous, inspissated meconium
- commonly seen in cystic fibrosis
- presents with abdominal distention and failure to pass meconium after birth
- treat with gastrografin (water-soluble) enema, surgical laparotomy if refractory

ID/CC   A **1-day-old** male infant is seen by a neonatologist for **failure to pass meconium** and persistent **bilious vomiting** after each feeding.

HPI   The infant is the first-born child of a healthy 40-year-old woman who had **polyhydramnios**. The child was born **premature** at 32 weeks' gestation and suffers from **Down's syndrome**.

PE   VS: normal. PE: **hypotonic** and mildly dehydrated with dry mucous membranes; flattened face, low-set ears, macroglossia, flattened nasal bridge, and **epicanthal folds** (all consistent with Down's syndrome); **abdomen distended** and tympanic to percussion; **visible peristalsis**.

Labs   CBC: normal. Lytes: hypokalemia; hyponatremia; hypochloremia. BUN slightly increased with normal creatinine (dehydration). ABGs: metabolic alkalosis (vomiting, loss of hydrochloric acid). Karyotype: trisomy 21.

Imaging   **[A]** XR, abdomen: dilatation of the gastric chamber (1) and proximal duodenum (2) with no air in the remainder of the bowel, producing the typical image ("double bubble"). **[B]** US,

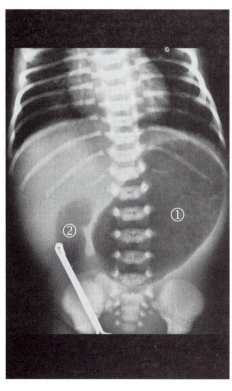

[A]

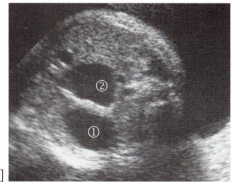

[B]

DUODENAL ATRESIA

fetal: a different case with dilated fluid-filled stomach (1) and duodenum (2). BE: normal (rule out malrotation).

Pathogenesis Duodenal atresia occurs as a result of failure of the second part of the duodenum to canalize during embryonic development. It is commonly associated with prematurity, **polyhydramnios**, and **Down's syndrome** and typically presents with **bilious vomiting** during the **first day of life**.

Epidemiology After the ileum, the duodenum is the most common site of congenital intestinal atresia.

Management **Restoration of fluid and electrolyte balance** is of paramount importance. **Nasogastric suction** is instituted to decompress the abdomen and relieve signs of obstruction (> 40 cc of residual gastric material is diagnostic of obstruction), followed by **surgical repair**. Treatment usually involves a side-to-side duodeno-duodenostomy with a protective tube gastrostomy.

ID/CC	A **1-day-old** male infant presents with **yellowing of the skin and eyes** and **generalized swelling of the body** (ANASARCA).

HPI The **amniotic fluid** was **yellow** and the **placenta was enlarged** at the time of delivery. The child's mother is an otherwise-healthy 24-year-old **white** female who is **Rh negative**. This is her **second child**.

PE VS: tachycardia. PE: generalized edema; marked **jaundice** with **yellow vernix; petechiae** on legs and arms; muscular **hypotonia** and **lethargy** (severe disease); decreased breath sounds in left lung field (due to pleural effusion); abdominal exam reveals **hepatosplenomegaly** (compensatory extramedullary erythropoiesis) and ascites.

Labs CBC/PBS: **anemia** (7 mg/dL); thrombocytopenia; polychromasia; **nucleated erythrocytes** (ERYTHROBLASTS); **direct Coombs' test positive** (child's serum); **indirect Coombs' test positive** (antibodies in maternal blood); anti-Rh agglutinins positive in infant's blood. LFTs: **increased indirect bilirubin** (due to hemolysis).

Imaging CXR: mild left pleural effusion. KUB: ascites.

Pathogenesis Erythroblastosis fetalis can occur in **Rh-positive fetuses** of previously **sensitized Rh-negative mothers**. During the first pregnancy, Rh-positive fetal erythrocytes reach the maternal circulation (in the third trimester and during delivery) and stimulate antibody production against the Rh antigen. In subsequent pregnancies, these maternal antibodies pass to the fetus via the placenta and destroy fetal erythrocytes (if Rh positive). This hemolysis leads to compensatory overproduction of nucleated erythrocytes (ERYTHROBLASTS). The clinical spectrum of disease ranges from mild anemia and jaundice to erythroblastosis fetalis to hydrops fetalis. ABO incompatibility rarely leads to erythroblastosis fetalis.

Epidemiology More common in **whites. Predisposing factors** include previous Rh-positive pregnancy or maternal exposure to fetal blood during C-section, abortion, or amniocentesis.

Management Treat with **phenobarbital** (reduces bilirubin) prior to delivery. If the mother's Rh Ab titer is ≥ 1:16, perform paired amniocentesis. Perform **intrauterine transfusion** if fetal hematocrit drops below 30%. **Induce labor** in the presence of previous severe hemolytic disease, if hydrops is seen on ultrasound, or in cases of fetal pulmonary maturity. Perform **exchange transfusion** in the presence of jaundice at birth, kernicterus, bilirubin > 15 mg/dL, a rise in indirect bilirubin > 0.5 mg/dL/hr or cord bilirubin > 4.0 mg/dL, methemalbuminemia, or anemia < 45 HT. Cross-match type O Rh-negative whole blood and exchange. **Phototherapy** may be used in ABO disease if bilirubin > 10 and may be used in Rh disease in conjunction with transfusion. Late anemia may occur after days or weeks and is more frequent in Rh than in ABO incompatibility. To prevent this complication, administer **RhoGAM** intramuscularly immediately after delivery for Rh-negative mothers (prevents sensitization). Also give for ectopic pregnancy and induced or spontaneous abortion.

Complications Complications include stillbirths, hydrops fetalis, and **kernicterus** that may proceed to potentially fatal brain damage (bilirubin deposition in basal ganglia). The risk of kernicterus increases with hypoglycemia, drugs that displace bilirubin from albumin (sulfisoxazole), acidosis, hypoxia, hypothermia, and indirect bilirubin > 20 mg/dL. Sequelae include mental retardation, cerebral palsy, and sensorineural deafness.

ID/CC A 32-week-gestation (**premature**) male infant has bluish skin (CYANOSIS) after delivery by cesarean section.

HPI His mother had **third-trimester bleeding** and uterine contractions that did not stop with rest or medical management. The child's **Apgar score was low** at 5 minutes (6).

PE VS: marked **tachypnea**; tachycardia; **hypothermia; hypotension**. PE: infant weighs 1.85 kg; uses **accessory muscles** of respiration; **nasal flaring; intercostal** and supraclavicular **retractions; cyanosis** of lips and fingers; **grunting; tubular breath sounds and rales**.

Labs ABGs: **hypoxemia; hypercapnia**; mixed respiratory/metabolic (LACTIC) acidosis. **Decreased lecithin-to-sphingomyelin (L/S) ratio in amniotic fluid**.

Imaging **[A]** CXR: indistinct diaphragm; **reticular pulmonary infiltrates bilaterally** and diffuse **atelectasis** with increased lung field opacification and **air bronchograms** (signs may not be present in first 6 to 12 hours). **[B]** CXR: normal premature neonatal chest film for comparison.

Pathogenesis Hyaline membrane disease is caused by a **deficiency of surfactant** (lipoprotein produced by type II pneumocytes, which decreases surface tension and stabilizes alveoli) that results in atelectasis. **Atelectasis** and **decreased compliance** lead in turn to greatly increased effort to expand the lungs, with subsequent respiratory failure, as well as to a very low functional residual capacity, hypoventilation, pulmonary vasoconstriction, **shunting, hypoxia, cyanosis**, and acidosis. Presents at birth or shortly thereafter.

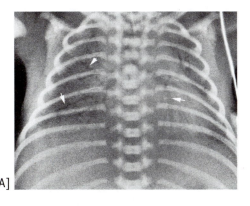
[A]

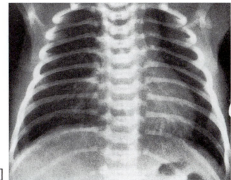
[B]

HYALINE MEMBRANE DISEASE

Epidemiology	The most common cause of respiratory distress in **premature infants**; incidence is 5% at 35 to 37 weeks' gestational age (GA) and > 50% at 26 to 28 weeks' GA. Associated with **cesarean births, infants of diabetic mothers, fetal distress**, and **obstetrical bleeding**.
Management	Intubation, **ventilatory support; fluid, acid-base**, and **electrolyte balance; antibiotics** if infection is suspected. Give **betamethasone** to nondiabetic pregnant women to increase fetal lung maturity; **surfactant** in premature infants. Infants generally improve 3 to 7 days after onset.
Complications	Complications often stem from supportive care: umbilical catheterization predisposes to infection and thrombosis; oxygen and pressure from ventilators may lead to **bronchopulmonary dysplasia; necrotizing enterocolitis; delayed closure of PDA** results from hypoxia, acidosis, and immaturity.
Atlas Link	U C V 1 PG-BC-083

ID/CC A **4-week-old male** infant is brought to the pediatrician because he has been **regurgitating** his food and has been having occasional bouts of vomiting for the past week.

HPI The infant continues to have a **voracious appetite**. Earlier that day he presented with **nonbilious projectile vomiting** both during and immediately after feeding.

PE VS: moderate tachycardia. PE: **lethargic** and mildly **dehydrated; low weight for age**; abdomen soft and flat; after nasogastric tube gastric emptying, 2-cm, firm, nontender, motile **olive-shaped mass** palpable in right upper quadrant; **peristalsis visible**.

Labs CBC: increased hematocrit (hemoconcentration secondary to dehydration). Lytes: **hypokalemia**; hyponatremia; **hypochloremia**. ABGs: metabolic alkalosis (due to loss of hydrochloric acid).

Imaging **[A]** UGI (with barium or water-soluble media): enlargement of the stomach chamber with increased peristalsis and delayed emptying with **string sign (1)** (narrowing and elongation of the pyloric canal). **[B]** US: **identification of hypertrophied muscle** (pyloric muscle thickness > 4 mm).

Pathogenesis Hypertrophic pyloric stenosis is idiopathic. Longitudinal and circular muscle fibers in the distal stomach and pyloric region are hypertrophied. This results in gastric outlet obstruction, poor feeding, abdominal distention after feeding, and vomiting. The vomiting progresses in frequency and force, ultimately leading to projectile vomiting. Vomit may contain blood but generally does not contain bile (obstruction proximal to the ampulla of Vater).

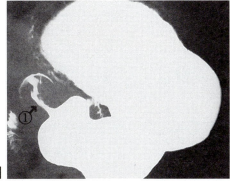

[A]

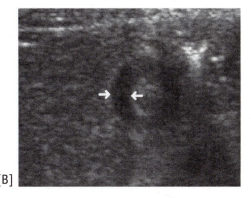

[B]

HYPERTROPHIC PYLORIC STENOSIS

Epidemiology	Relatively common cause of vomiting (1 in 500 births). More common in **male** and **full-term** infants. Higher risk in monozygotic twins. Onset of symptoms is usually during the **second or third week** of life.
Management	Perform **nasogastric tube** decompression; rehydrate and correct electrolyte imbalances. The definitive treatment is **Ramstedt pyloromyotomy**.
Complications	Hypokalemic, hypochloremic metabolic alkalosis (tetany), reflux esophagitis, weight loss and starvation, dehydration, unconjugated hyperbilirubinemia with jaundice (increased enterohepatic circulation), aspiration pneumonia, gastritis with bleeding (stasis), and learning disabilities if period of inanition was prolonged.

ID/CC A **3-day-old** infant **delivered prematurely** develops **abdominal distention, lethargy, bilious vomiting, feeding intolerance**, and **bright red blood per rectum** (HEMATOCHEZIA).

HPI He is the first-born child of an apparently healthy mother who had presented with **amnionitis**. The child weighed 1.95 kg.

PE VS: **hypothermia** with temperature instability; **bradycardia; hypotension**. PE: **lethargic** and icteric with periods of apnea; abdomen **distended and tympanic** with signs of **rigidity; absent bowel sounds**; marked rebound tenderness (peritonitis); **abdominal wall discoloration and "loopy" appearance**.

Labs CBC: **polycythemia** (Hb 17.1); **marked leukocytosis** (may show neutropenia in severe septicemia); **thrombocytopenia**. Blood cultures yield *Escherichia coli* and *Klebsiella*. ABGs: **metabolic acidosis**.

Imaging **[A]** CXR: a different case demonstrating free subdiaphragmatic air (PNEUMOPERITONEUM) (due to hollow viscus perforation). **[B]** KUB: edema of bowel wall; **pneumatosis intestinalis** (due to intramural gas); **intrahepatic portal venous gas** (late sign) and air-fluid levels may also be seen. BE is contraindicated (due to risk of perforation).

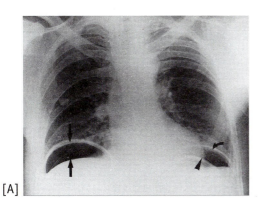
[A]

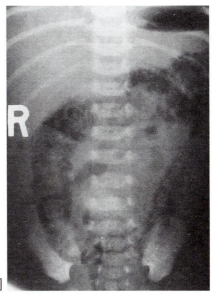
[B]

NECROTIZING ENTEROCOLITIS

Pathogenesis	Necrotizing enterocolitis may be related to **ischemic insult** that damages the bowel lining and hampers mucus production, rendering the bowel susceptible to infection. Mucosal damage and colonization lead to intramural hemorrhage, mucosal edema, necrosis, ulceration, membrane formation, gangrene, and perforation. Associated with **prematurity**, polycythemia, congenital heart disease, umbilical catheterization, broad-spectrum antibiotics, birth asphyxia, hypertonic milk, and rapid feeding.
Epidemiology	A **common neonatal GI emergency**. Onset is usually on the third day of life. Mortality rate is approximately 30%.
Management	**Supportive management** (in ICU) addresses temperature, ventilation, circulation, and anemia; **x-ray every 6 hours** for the first 12 to 48 hours (high perforation risk); institute **GI rest** (NPO, GI suction, peripheral parenteral nutrition); maintain fluid and electrolyte balance. **To control infection**, give carbenicillin/gentamicin or clindamycin/aminoglycosides for gram-negative organisms (risk of staphylococcal and *Candida* superinfection), vancomycin if clostridial. **Surgical resection** is required in the event of perforation, failure of medical therapy, abdominal wall cellulitis (erythema, warmth, induration), localized tenderness or mass > 12 hours, acidosis, or ascites.
Complications	**Strictures** may develop at the involved site; after resection, patients may develop **short bowel syndrome**.
Atlas Links	UCVI M-M1-033A, M-M1-033B, PG-M1-033

ID/CC	A 2-week-old female infant presents with **lethargy**, vomiting, and **feeding difficulties**.
HPI	Her mother states that the infant sometimes has **fever** and at other times has a **low temperature** (temperature instability).
PE	VS: low-grade **fever** (38.1°C); tachycardia; tachypnea. PE: inconsolable with high-pitched cry; **bulging fontanelle**; during examination, patient has episode of **projectile vomiting**.
Labs	CBC: **leukocytosis with neutrophilia**. Lytes: normal. BUN and creatinine normal. LP: **increased pressure; neutrophilic pleocytosis; low glucose; increased protein**. Gram-positive cocci in chains seen on Gram stain; culture grows **group B streptococcus**.
Imaging	CT/MR, brain: subtle meningeal thickening and enhancement.
Pathogenesis	The etiology of neonatal meningitis varies according to the time of onset. **Early-onset** infections (0 to 3 days) most frequently involve bacteremia with *Escherichia coli* or *Streptococcus agalactiae* (GROUP B STREP) and rarely lead to meningitis. **Late-onset** infections (14 to 28 days) are usually caused by **group B streptococcus** or *Listeria monocytogenes*, and **most progress** to meningitis. Early-onset infections are usually acquired perinatally from the maternal genital tract; late-onset infections are generally acquired from environmental (hospital or home) sources.
Management	For neonatal meningitis, give **ampicillin** (covers *Listeria*) with **gentamicin** or with **cefotaxime**. For *Haemophilus* or *Neisseria meningitides*, use ceftriaxone, cefuroxime, or ampicillin. For *Streptococcus pneumoniae*, treat with penicillin, ampicillin, or vancomycin. Corticosteroids are beneficial in *Haemophilus* meningitis.
Complications	Hydrocephalus, seizures, subdural effusion, brain abscess, and deafness.

NEONATAL MENINGITIS

ID/CC   A **5-day-old** female infant is seen for a **yellowish hue** in her eyes and skin (JAUNDICE). The problem was **first noted on the third day of life** and has since worsened.

HPI   The infant is the **first-born** child of an apparently healthy white couple (G6PD unlikely). She is on formula food (no breast-milk jaundice). The mother denies any drug intake in the third trimester, and there is no family history of jaundice.

PE   VS: normal. PE: **well developed** and in **no acute distress; no cataracts** (vs. galactosemia); moderate **icterus** of conjunctiva, sublingual mucosa, and skin; **stool normal color; no hepatosplenomegaly** (vs. Rh incompatibility) and **no masses** (vs. choledochal cyst).

Labs   CBC/PBS: normal hemoglobin; normal erythrocyte morphology; hemoglobin electrophoresis normal; reticulocyte count normal. **Coombs' test negative.** LFTs: **indirect bilirubin markedly elevated** (9 mg/dL); **direct bilirubin mildly elevated** (1 mg/dL). Mother and infant Rh positive.

Pathogenesis   Unconjugated bilirubin (major product of heme metabolism) is carried in the plasma by albumin and transported to the liver, where it is conjugated (by glucuronyl transferase) with glucuronic acid. Conjugated bilirubin is excreted with bile into the intestine, where gut flora convert it to urobilinogen. Urobilinogen returns to the liver via the enterohepatic circulation, is excreted in urine, or is converted to stercobilin and excreted in the feces. Neonates are predisposed to hyperbilirubinemia for reasons including (1) **increased bilirubin load** due to increased RBC mass and decreased RBC half-life, (2) **decreased** hepatic **glucuronyl transferase** activity, and (3) increased enterohepatic circulation and decreased conversion of bilirubin to urobilinogen (with subsequent reabsorption of bilirubin) because of decreased intestinal flora. Physiologic jaundice appears **after the first day**, peaks between the third and fifth day (more in prematures), and returns to normal in 2 weeks, with bilirubin that does not exceed 12 (15 in premature babies). The diagnosis is one of exclusion.

Epidemiology   More common in Asians. Predisposing factors include **prematurity, dehydration, and malnutrition, breastfeeding**, and maternal diabetes.

Management   Usually **no treatment** is needed. **Phototherapy** or **exchange transfusion** may be used if bilirubin rises rapidly. Maintain good hydration and nutrition.

PHYSIOLOGIC JAUNDICE OF NEWBORN

ID/CC	A **3-month-old male** infant cannot be awakened by his mother and has blue lips. When the paramedics arrive a few minutes later, it is clear that the child has been dead for at least 4 hours.
HPI	The infant was born **prematurely**. Both parents are 19-year-old **Native Americans** who live in an **inner-city** area. The **mother smoked during pregnancy and did not receive prenatal care**. On directed questioning, the parents state that the child had had an **unusual cry** lately, together with episodes of **apnea**. Last week he also had a **URI**.
PE	Autopsy showed petechiae on pericardial and pleural surfaces along with **gliosis of brainstem** and **hypertrophy of pulmonary smooth muscle** vasculature (long-existing hypoxia).
Labs	UA: toxicology screen negative.
Pathogenesis	Sudden infant death syndrome (SIDS) is defined as an **unexplained sudden death** that cannot be accounted for by any abnormality on autopsy. Recurrent or chronic hypoxia may be caused by an abnormality in autonomic cardiopulmonary regulation.
Epidemiology	SIDS occurs in 1 in 1,000 live births and is the **most common cause of death in infants younger than 1 year of age**. It most commonly occurs during sleep, at night, and in infants aged **2 to 4 months** (rare before 1 month and after 9 months). Risk factors include poor and nonwhite infants, mothers who smoke or who have a history of substance abuse, prematurity, and previous loss of an infant to SIDS.
Management	Provide **counseling** support for parents (for strong guilt feelings), continuing until and after parents decide to have a new baby. Impedance monitoring, performed at home for subsequent children as well as for children with apneic episodes, is warranted in some cases. Putting **infants to sleep on their back** and maternal smoking cessation (including prenatally) decrease SIDS risk.

SUDDEN INFANT DEATH SYNDROME

ID/CC	A 5-year-old boy presents with **malaise, periorbital edema, smoky-colored urine** (HEMATURIA), abdominal pain with vomiting, and mild **fever**.
HPI	Ten days ago he had a **throat infection** (due to a nephritogenic strain of *Streptococcus*), from which he recovered uneventfully.
PE	VS: **hypertension** (BP 140/90). PE: mild **pallor**; no cyanosis or jaundice; **palpebral edema**; tonsils inflamed but no exudate; regular rate and rhythm with no murmurs; no hepatosplenomegaly; **ankle edema** (2+); no skin rashes.
Labs	CBC: **anemia**; leukocytosis. **Increased ESR; increased BUN and creatinine**. ABGs: **metabolic acidosis**. Lytes: **hyperkalemia**. UA: **RBCs and RBC casts**; leukocyturia and proteinuria; hemoglobinuria. **C3 and total hemolytic complement** (CH_{50}) **low** (almost always); **increased ASO titer** (recent streptococcal infection); throat culture does not reveal *Streptococcus* (only 4% positive rate); ANA negative; DNase antibody titer high.
Imaging	CXR/KUB: normal.
Pathogenesis	Poststreptococcal glomerulonephritis is an immune complex disease that is usually caused by group A β-hemolytic streptococcus types 12 and 49. It occurs **7 to 14 days after strep infection**. Pathogenesis may be related to the deposition of streptococcal **antigen-antibody complexes in the glomeruli**, followed by inflammation due to complement activation. Electron microscopy reveals **electron-dense humps** (immune complexes) on the epithelial side of the glomerular basement membrane. Immunofluorescence demonstrates a granular pattern of immunoglobulin deposition.
Epidemiology	Common childhood nephritis; affects preschool and school-age children. May be isolated or occur in epidemics. Occurs after tonsillitis, pharyngitis, skin infection, and scarlet fever. A history of strep infection is found in 95% of cases.
Management	**Treat infection with penicillin** for 10 days to prevent spread of nephritogenic strain (erythromycin if allergic). Diet high in carbohydrates and low in protein, sodium, potassium, and water. Treat **renal** and **cardiac failure** with peritoneal dialysis. Resolution may take 6 to 12 months (microscopic hematuria up to 1 year).

POSTSTREPTOCOCCAL GLOMERULONEPHRITIS

Complications   Cardiac failure, hypertensive encephalopathy (vomiting, severe headache, convulsions, visual disturbances), uremia, acute pulmonary edema, and chronic glomerulonephritis.

MINICASE 333: ALPORT'S DISEASE

An X-linked genetic connective tissue disease
- presents with hematuria, deafness, renal failure, and cataracts
- no known treatment is available

MINICASE 334: TESTICULAR DYSGENESIS

A developmental defect causing seminiferous tubule degeneration and absent müllerian structures
- presents with ambiguous external genitalia, maldescended dysgenetic testes, and usually bilateral inguinal swelling
- treat with gonadectomy, hormone replacement therapy

ID/CC	A **3-year-old child** is admitted with an **abdominal mass** that was detected on routine exam.
HPI	The child is **asymptomatic**, has no history of hematuria, has never been diagnosed as hypertensive, and does not suffer from any obvious congenital malformation. Neither parent reports any familial disease.
PE	VS: normal BP. PE: appears normal; weight and height normal for age; abdomen appears distended; large, **firm, nontender intra-abdominal mass** palpated toward the right, not crossing midline.
Labs	CBC/UA: normal. LFTs: normal. Mass biopsy reveals sheets of **small oval cells with scant cytoplasm** and primitive glomerular and tubular structures occasionally seen; urinary vanillylmandelic acid (VMA) levels normal (to rule out neuroblastoma).
Imaging	US, abdomen: a massive **intra-abdominal tumor arising out of the right kidney**. CT, abdomen (used to define extent of local invasion and involvement of inferior vena cava): normal IVC.
Pathogenesis	Wilms' tumor is a neoplastic disease of unknown etiology. Karyotypic abnormalities, particularly deletions of the short arm of chromosome 11, may be etiologically important. The tumor results from **neoplastic embryonal renal cells** of the metanephros. Both Wilms' tumor and retinoblastoma are postulated to evolve through two distinct "hits" to the host genome. There is prezygotic (germ-line) inheritance of the first hit. The postzygotic (somatic) mutation, the second hit, induces malignancy in the tissue rendered susceptible by the first hit.
Epidemiology	Wilms' tumor is the **second most common abdominal neoplasm** in children (behind neuroblastoma) and occurs with equal frequency in boys and girls. The usual age of diagnosis is between 4 months and 6 years, with the **median age** being about **3 years**. Ten percent of patients have bilateral Wilms' tumors. Children with sporadic aniridia, hemihypertrophy, and GU abnormalities are at increased risk for Wilms' tumor. **WAGR syndrome** is characterized by Wilms' tumor, aniridia, ambiguous genitalia, and mental retardation.
Management	Requires **surgical resection** of the primary tumor and any lymph nodes or selected metastases. **Radiotherapy** is used to treat

WILMS' TUMOR

residual local disease and selected metastatic foci. **Chemotherapy varies in duration and intensity depending on the stage and histology, but regimens usually include actinomycin D and vincristine.**

ID/CC	A 4-year-old boy is evaluated for **difficulty running**.
HPI	The mother states that her son was one of the last children to walk, adding that he is **unable to keep up with his friends**. He is also **unable to jump or hop normally**, and he **climbs stairs one foot at a time**. He must use his hands when standing up from the floor (GOWERS' MANEUVER).
PE	VS: normal. PE: **positive Gowers' sign** (weakness of lower back and pelvic girdle musculature); **enlarged firm, rubbery calves** (PSEUDOHYPERTROPHY); waddling (TRENDELENBURG) gait.
Labs	**Serum CK elevated to 20 to 100 times normal**. EMG: myopathy. Muscle biopsy shows fibers of varying size with replacement by fat and connective tissue; **dystrophin deficiency**.
Pathogenesis	Duchenne's muscular dystrophy (DMD), or **pseudohypertrophic muscular dystrophy**, is **an X-linked recessive disorder** caused by **mutations in the dystrophin gene, a gene that codes for a sarcolemmal protein**. DMD is characterized by **profound progressive muscle weakness** that is **first observed in the proximal muscles**. Patients are generally delayed in their walking and demonstrate significant difficulty running and jumping. At a young age, their calf muscles hypertrophy, but the hypertrophic muscle is eventually replaced by fat and connective tissue. As the children age, they require braces to walk and eventually are confined to a wheelchair. Additionally, boys suffer from chest wall deformities, further impairing their respiratory performance and placing them at risk for fatal pulmonary infections by 16 to 18 years of age.
Epidemiology	DMD has an incidence of approximately 3 in 10,000 and arises **almost exclusively in boys**.
Management	**Prednisone** may slow disease progression. Patients should also receive **orthotic and orthopedic treatments**. Parents should be referred for **genetic counseling**.
Complications	Intellectual impairment (mean IQ approximately 85), kyphoscoliosis, cardiomyopathy, cardiac arrhythmias, CHF, pulmonary infections, and respiratory failure.
Atlas Links	⬚ⓊⒸⓋ2 **PED-049**　　ⓊⒸⓋ1 PM-BC-086, PG-BC-086

NEUROLOGY

DUCHENNE'S MUSCULAR DYSTROPHY

ID/CC   A **7-year-old boy** is seen for a **limp in his right leg** of about 3 months' duration with no apparent cause.

HPI   He also complains of **groin pain** that **radiates to the inner thigh** (pain in slipped capital femoral epiphysis is referred to the medial knee). He denies any trauma or recent infections.

PE   VS: normal. PE: well developed and well nourished; **right leg shorter** than left; **tenderness and muscle spasticity** over right **hip joint**; decreased range of motion on abduction and internal rotation of affected hip.

Labs   Unremarkable.

Imaging   **[A]** XR, hip: small femoral head epiphysis with increased density (SCLEROSIS). Partial vs. total collapse of the femoral head can also be seen on radiographs in advanced stages of disease. **[B]** XR, hip: a different case with severe flattening and sclerosis of the right femoral head (1). MR (preferred for making diagnosis):

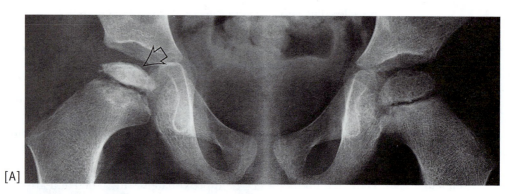

[A]

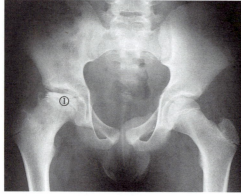

[B]

marrow edema and fracture line in the femoral head. Nuc: abnormal uptake in the femoral head.

Pathogenesis   Legg–Calve–Perthes disease is an idiopathic type of avascular necrosis of bone. The process is self-limited for a period of up to 3 years. Roughly half of all patients recover fully with bone revascularization; half will have permanent hip deformity.

Epidemiology   **More common in boys** than in girls; primarily affects children **between 3 and 12 years**.

Management   Weight bearing may be permitted with the use of a **Petrie walking cast** in which the joint is braced so that proper remodeling of bone can occur (in **abduction and medial rotation**). Moderate to severe cases are treated with **acetabular** or **femoral osteotomy**.

ID/CC A 1-year-old **girl** is evaluated for a **limp**.

HPI She has just begun to walk, and the parents noticed a marked **deficit in her left hip and leg**. She is the **first-born child** of a healthy couple of **Navajo Indian** origin. Directed questioning discloses that the child was born in a **breech presentation**.

PE Asymmetry of gluteal folds (present in 40% of normal newborns); **inability to passively abduct the left flexed hip to 90 degrees**; leg in external rotation; lordosis and **waddling gait**; abduction of affected thigh causes palpable click as femoral head returns to acetabulum (ORTOLANI'S SIGN); with hips kept in 90-degree flexion, level of knee height is lower in affected side (GALEAZZI'S SIGN with unilateral involvement); hip falls to unaffected side when child stands on foot of affected side (TRENDELENBURG'S SIGN).

Labs Normal.

Imaging **[A]** A different case with bilateral femoral head dislocation and shallow **dysplastic acetabula** (1). **[B]** XR, pelvis: a different case with delayed appearance of the femoral ossification center (1) on the right side. (X-rays are not useful before 6 weeks of age. US is therefore more sensitive for diagnosis in neonates, since the ossification center is not seen on radiographs.)

Pathogenesis Congenital dislocation of the hip is an abnormal relationship between the head of the femur and the acetabular articular surface due to mechanical defects (breech presentation, first born, oligohydramnios) that produce instability leading to dislocation of the hip joint. Also called **developmental dysplasia of the hip**. Dislocation may be partial or complete.

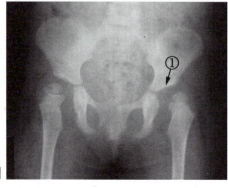

[A]

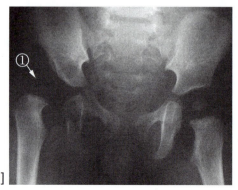

[B]

Epidemiology Occurs in 1 in 1,000 births, with a higher incidence found in Navajo Indians and a low incidence among blacks. Affects **females** more frequently than males and first-born children more than subsequent pregnancies. Occurs more frequently on the left side and is bilateral in one-fifth of all cases. It is associated with **breech** presentations, congenital torticollis, and spina bifida.

Management The key to correct management of congenital dislocation of the hip lies in **early diagnosis**; the sooner it is diagnosed the better, and screening should continue for at least 1 year following diagnosis. The newborn exam is the most important one from a diagnostic perspective, but follow-up exams are also needed to detect later-onset congenital hip dislocation. In children younger than 3 months of age, **a Frejka pillow, a Pavlik harness, or a spica cast** is used for 3 months to keep the hip flexed and abducted with the femoral head in place. Forced abduction is undesirable owing to the risk of aseptic necrosis of the femoral head. In children older than 6 months, an adductor myotomy or elongation is needed for reduction, followed by a spica cast for longer periods. In children older than 18 months, osteotomy and open reduction are needed. Success is inversely proportional to age at diagnosis.

Complications Flattening of the acetabular articular surface with osteoarthritis of the joint, aseptic necrosis of the femoral head, swaying (unilateral involvement) or waddling (bilateral involvement) gait, and limping.

Atlas Links UCV2 PED-051A, PED-051B

ID/CC	A 6-year-old child is brought to the ER by his parents with acute **pain and deformity** of his left arm (due to fracture) that began during warm-up exercises for physical education class (minor trauma).
HPI	The child has sustained **four fractures** in the last two **2 years**.
PE	VS: normal. PE: short for age; **blue sclerae**; corneal opacities; keratoconus; partial **conduction deafness** in both ears (most common after 10 years of age); **abnormal teeth** (DENTINOGENESIS IMPERFECTA); hand and finger joints show **increased elasticity; kyphosis and scoliosis present**.
Labs	Unremarkable.
Imaging	XR: generalized **osteopenia with radiolucency of long bones**; wormian bones in the skull; vertebrae appear flattened; **poorly healed old fractures**; acute **left humeral fracture**; significant bony bowing and angular deformity may be present.
Pathogenesis	Also called **brittle bone disease**, osteogenesis imperfecta is an **autosomal-dominant** disorder of connective tissue characterized by a mutation in the gene that codes for **type I collagen**, resulting in abnormal collagen synthesis and deficient ossification and **frequent fractures** in children. Patients frequently present with **blue sclerae and conduction deafness**, abnormal platelet function, and hyperkinetic circulation.
Epidemiology	A rare disorder. Fractures generally do not occur before the first year of life.

OSTEOGENESIS IMPERFECTA

Management   Treatment is **supportive**, with orthopedic treatment of fractures and deformities along with physiotherapy and rehabilitation. Growth hormone and calcitonin are investigational. Ascorbic acid and calcium are usually given. Prevention through **genetic counseling** is necessary, since this is an autosomal-dominant disorder.

Complications   **Skull fracture during delivery**; multiple fractures and **recurrent joint dislocations**.

Atlas Link   UCV2 **PED-052**

ID/CC	A **1-year-old** boy is brought to the emergency room with a swollen left thigh.
HPI	The mother, who appears very concerned, **states that the child fell from the bed**. She is a divorcée who is now living with a new boyfriend.
PE	Child looks **apprehensive** and begins to cry even when touched gently; **retinal hemorrhages** present; tender swelling seen over left thigh; **multiple bruises seen over body** in various stages of resolution (mother suspects a clotting defect).
Labs	Coagulation profile normal.
Imaging	XR, left thigh: spiral fracture of the femur. Skeletal survey: **old fractures** in the humerus, both tibia, and ribs, seen in **different stages of healing** (highly suggestive of child abuse). Bone density normal (metabolically normal bones).
Pathogenesis	**Injuries intentionally perpetrated by a caretaker that result in morbidity or mortality constitute physical abuse.** Failure to provide a child with appropriate food, clothing, medical care, schooling, and a safe environment constitutes neglect. Instances that should arouse suspicion of abuse include cuts and bruises in low-trauma areas such as the buttocks or back, fractures that occur before ambulation, multiple fractures in different stages of healing in metabolically normal bones (thereby excluding osteogenesis imperfecta), metaphyseal fractures, **multiple bruises over the body in the absence of any bleeding disorder**, burns, injury that is inconsistent with the stated history, unexplained delay in obtaining appropriate medical care, or **retinal hemorrhages** that result from vigorous shaking ("shaken baby syndrome").
Epidemiology	Almost half of the children who receive medical attention as a result of physical abuse are younger than 1 year, and the vast majority are preschoolers. Parents, mothers' boyfriends, babysitters, and stepparents are the most frequent perpetrators. Mortality is 5%.
Management	Health care workers are **required by law to report any suspicion** of child abuse or neglect to state protection agencies. Physicians are not liable for any damages even if the abuse is disproved later. Suitable orthopedic treatment for injuries.
Atlas Link	⬜️𝐔𝐂𝐕𝟐 **PED-053**

CHILD ABUSE—PHYSICAL

ID/CC A 10-year-old boy presents with chest congestion, **cough, difficulty breathing, and wheezing**.

HPI His symptoms started 4 days ago when he caught a **cold**. He is **allergic to cats and pollen** and had **eczema** during infancy as well as **allergic rhinitis**. He has had repeated attacks of wheezing over the years (asthma), one of which required hospitalization. His **mother and maternal uncle** suffer from severe **asthma**.

PE VS: slight fever; **tachypnea**; tachycardia. PE: **dyspnea** with increased respiratory effort; **nasal mucosa** boggy and **pale** (due to allergy); uses **accessory muscles** of respiration; **expiratory wheezes and high-pitched sibilant rhonchi** heard throughout lung fields; **prolongation of expiration; hyperresonance** to percussion.

Labs CBC: leukocytosis with lymphocytosis (viral infection) and **eosinophilia** (allergic component). Increased serum IgE. ABGs: **respiratory alkalosis, hypocarbia, and hypoxemia** (in severe cases, CO_2 retention [respiratory acidosis]). PFTs: increased total lung capacity and residual volume; **decreased FEV_1/FVC** (reversible with β-agonists).

Imaging CXR: lung **hyperinflation** with flattened diaphragm; peribronchial cuffing and linear atelectasis in both bases.

Pathogenesis Asthma is characterized by **episodic airway hyperreactivity** and inflammation. It may be intrinsic or initiated by an **allergen** (type I hypersensitivity reaction). One observes reversible constriction of airway smooth muscle, hypersecretion of mucus, edema, inflammatory cell (particularly mast cell) infiltration, and epithelial desquamation. In atopic asthma, **a biphasic response** is frequently observed. An acute phase is marked by immediate hypersensitivity and mast cell degranulation, with return toward baseline within 1 hour. Recurrences, which are characterized by more severe airway obstruction, arise 3 to 8 hours after initial exposure.

Epidemiology Affects 5% of U.S. population. May be **extrinsic** (allergic; best prognosis) or **intrinsic** (idiosyncratic; no hypersensitivity). Fifty percent of patients outgrow asthma after puberty. Associated with hay fever, rhinitis, urticaria, aspirin sensitivity (nasal polyps), eczema, and family history.

Management Acute management includes **oxygen, bronchodilators** (β-agonists or anticholinergics), and **corticosteroids**; subcutaneous adrenaline in severe instances. Chronic management involves avoidance of allergens, regularly inhaled bronchodilators or steroids, systemic steroids, immunotherapy, cromolyn, or theophylline (check blood levels). Start **anti-inflammatory agents (cromolyn, steroids)** if the patient is symptomatic more than 2 times a week or has nocturnal symptoms more than 2 times a month. Leukotriene antagonists can be used as adjuncts.

Complications Pneumothorax, pulsus paradoxus (very severe asthma), orthopnea, and respiratory failure.

ID/CC	A **2-year-old girl** is brought to the pediatrician with **swelling and pain in her right knee of 3 months' duration**.
HPI	Yesterday she developed a **rash** and became fatigued. Her mother has also noticed **"redness" of the eyes** (due to uveitis).
PE	VS: normal. PE: micrognathia; slit-lamp exam shows **uveitis**; right knee swollen, erythematous, and tender to palpation with **limitation of passive and active movements**.
Labs	CBC: normocytic, normochromic anemia. **ESR elevated; ANA positive; rheumatoid factor (RF) negative** (RF may be positive in polyarticular type).
Imaging	XR, knee: soft tissue swelling; osteopenia.
Pathogenesis	Juvenile rheumatoid arthritis (JRA) is idiopathic in nature but has an immune component. Articular involvement of **at least one joint for at least 6 weeks** in a child **younger than 16 years** is necessary for diagnosis. Several infectious agents, including rubella, herpesvirus, and EBV, have been implicated. JRA is divided into three types: pauciarticular, polyarticular, and systemic. The **pauciarticular form** is the most common variety and generally presents with involvement of one joint, usually the knee. The ankles are also commonly affected. It is associated with HLA-DR5 and uveitis and is more common in girls. The **polyarticular form** is associated with HLA-DR4 and involves five or more joints with symmetrical involvement; there is a female predisposition, and rheumatoid factor is usually negative. **Systemic disease** (STILL'S DISEASE) is associated with high, spiking fever, rash, leukocytosis with neutrophilia, splenomegaly, and markedly elevated ESR. ANA and rheumatoid factor are usually negative.
Epidemiology	More common in **girls**; onset is before 16 years of age. Half a million patients are diagnosed with JRA each year in the United States. There are two peaks of incidence: from 1 to 3 years and from 8 to 12 years.
Management	**Aspirin** for pauciarticular variety unless chickenpox or flu is suspected (risk of Reye's syndrome). Polyarticular or systemic-onset disease may require **chloroquine, methotrexate**, or other **immunosuppressive agents**. If carditis or hemolytic anemia is present, **steroids** may be used.
Complications	Chronicity, recurrence, disability, chronic uveitis, and progression to ankylosing spondylitis, iridocyclitis, and blindness.

JUVENILE RHEUMATOID ARTHRITIS

ID/CC	A 14-year-old girl is found lying semiconscious in her room by her mother.
HPI	The mother found a suicide note and an empty **pesticide** bottle lying in the room. The girl **vomited and passed loose stools** several times while being brought to the hospital.
PE	VS: **bradycardia** (HR 50). PE: drowsy and dehydrated; breath smells strongly of a **pesticide; pupils are pinpoint** with **hypersalivation; lacrimation**.
Labs	Red cell cholinesterase activity level < 25% of normal.
Pathogenesis	Organophosphates and carbamates (OPCs) are widely used as pesticides. They **inhibit the enzyme acetylcholinesterase**, decreasing the breakdown of acetylcholine at cholinergic synapses. Whereas the organophosphates may cause permanent inhibition of the enzyme, carbamates have a transient and reversible effect. Many of these agents are well **absorbed through intact skin**.
Epidemiology	Individuals may be exposed accidentally while working with or transporting the chemicals or as a result of accidental or intentional ingestion.
Management	As an initial step in management, it is important to immediately remove all contaminated clothing and wash all exposed areas with **soap and water**. Specific therapy includes administration of **atropine and pralidoxime (2-PAM)**. Atropine is not a pharmacologic antidote but can reverse excessive muscarinic stimulation, thereby **alleviating bradycardia, abdominal cramps, bronchospasm, and hypersalivation** (it does not reverse muscle weakness). All patients should also be given pralidoxime, since it restores the enzyme acetylcholinesterase. In those who go untreated, the organophosphates binding to acetylcholinesterase may become irreversible (the so-called aging effect). Because carbamates have a transient effect, pralidoxime therapy is not needed.

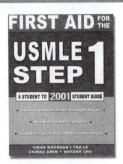
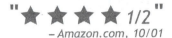
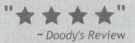
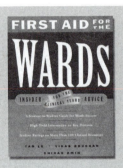
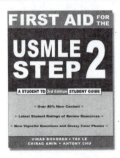
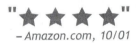
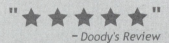
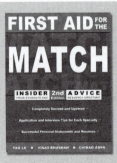